Hidden Aspects of Palliative Care

Other titles available in the Palliative Care series:

Why is it so difficult to die? by Brian Nyatanga

Fundamental Aspects of Palliative Care Nursing by Robert Becker and Richard Gamlin

Palliative Care for the Child with Malignant Disease edited by The West Midlands Paediatric Macmillan Team

Palliative Care for the Primary Care Team by Eileen Palmer and John Howarth

Palliative Care for People with Learning Disabilities edited by Sue Read

Series editor: Brian Nyatanga

Hidden Aspects of Palliative Care

edited by

Brian Nyatanga and Maxine Astley-Pepper

Quay Books
MA Healthcare Limited

Quay Books Division, MA Healthcare Limited, St Jude's Church, Dulwich Road,
London SE24 0PB

British Library Cataloguing-in-Publication Data
A catalogue record is available for this book

Printed in the UK by Cromwell Press, Trowbridge, Wiltshire

Contents

List of contributors

Maxine Astley-Pepper is Macmillan Senior Lecturer at the University of Central England in Birmingham.

Janine Birley is Lead Cancer Nurse Specialist at the Rotherham NHS Trust in South Yorkshire.

Heather Davies is Lecturer at the University of West of England in Bristol.

Craig Gannon is Consultant in Palliative Medicine at the Princess Alice Hospice in Esher and North Surrey PCT.

Nic Hughes is Macmillan Lecturer at the University of Leeds.

Wilf MacSherry is Senior Lecturer in the Faculty of Health and Social Care at the University of Hull.

Gwyneth Morgan is Senior Lecturer at the University of Central England.

Eileen Mullard is Macmillan Lecturer at the University of Leeds.

Brian Nyatanga is Macmillan Senior Lecturer at the University of Central England in Birmingham.

Liz Searle is Head of Palliative Care Services at Sue Ryder Care.

Helen Walsh is Macmillan Senior Nurse at Tyolwen Hospice at Morrison Hospital, Swansea.

Foreword

It is with great pleasure that I write the foreword to this new addition to the growing literature addressing issues in palliative care.

If there is one certainty in this life, it is that we shall all die. It is far less certain that we shall all be able to choose where we spend our last days, that we shall all be cared for by knowledgeable and skilled experts, and that the whole range of our anxieties and concerns will be taken into account as our care is planned.

However, the current high-profile of 'end-of-life' care and palliative care in general provides a very real opportunity to build on the successes and developments of the past and make some real changes for the future. This book will encourage new thinking and approaches to palliative care, not just for healthcare professionals.

It is not so long ago that symptom control, care of the dying, and support for the bereaved were fairly low priorities on the care agenda. Thankfully, there have been fundamental changes in culture, perceptions, and in the design and development of services. The frightening phrase 'terminal care' has been replaced by the more acceptable, but often little understood, 'palliative care'.

Cancer care has led the way in promoting the importance of palliative care, not just at the end of life, but throughout the experience of the disease — from the point that a diagnosis raises anxieties and distress, through the management of symptoms associated with the disease or its treatment, to the support of patients and families when cure is not longer an option.

Macmillan Cancer Relief has contributed to the expansion of expertise through the innovative use of pump-priming monies, the establishment of posts for nurses, doctors and consultants in palliative care, and a range of other professionals and services. As we move into the twenty-first century, we have unprecedented opportunities to translate this learning into other disease specialties and areas of care.

But there are also opportunities to extend the breadth and depth of palliative-care expertise. It is a relatively new art and science. Knowledge is growing, skills are being learnt, and standards are being raised as specialists share their expertise with generalists who are providing day-to-day care for a wide range of people. Excellence in palliative care will be delivered best through effective team work: where teams are made up not just of healthcare professionals, but also of experts from social care, lay people, and patients and carers themselves. As the most acute needs are assessed, identified and met, some of the less talked about 'hidden' aspects of care will be revealed. Anxieties and concerns that had previously not been considered can be acknowledged and shared, and interventions can be developed to manage them.

In Victorian times, sex was a taboo topic for polite conversation. Today, death and dying seem to have taken its place. Many people are uncomfortable talking about death or end-of-life care. It is one sure way of stopping a dinner-table conversation or of having the subject rapidly changed. It is time to change this situation and to allow open and honest acknowledgment that death is something that will affect us all and that we can all play a part in ensuring that, when it comes, death will be handled with the comprehensive approach that we have come to expect in other areas of care.

The topics discussed in this new book open up some of those difficult and often hidden areas. The crucial importance of team work is not in dispute. However, when truth-telling is incomplete, and professionals write one thing in their notes and say another thing to the patients and their families, then trust is betrayed. This is not a sound basis for care. How often is the emotional load of caring in a palliative situation addressed? Do we really support our staff sufficiently? And what of the person who is dying? Do we really understand the 'suffering' that he or she is experiencing, or consider the depths of their isolation? Expressing sexuality and love in the face of overwhelming disease and emotional distress do not often feature in a standard assessment — so how can discussion be encouraged if the problem is hidden?

The old adage 'a problem shared is a problem halved' could be applied to these hidden aspects of palliative care. All members of the team need to develop an awareness and sensitivity to the range of topics suggested in this text. Knowing about them is the first step towards being able to encourage and support a change in behaviour and practice. This new text will play its part in the development and expansion of palliative-care services to the ultimate benefit of all those who need them. There is no benefit to the patient if the different aspects in palliative care remain hidden.

Dame Gill Oliver
Director of Service Development
Macmillan Cancer Relief

Introduction

This book offers eclectic perspectives on hidden aspects of palliative and cancer care for all healthcare professionals. These include practical, clinical and philosophical perspectives for students, practitioners and academics alike. Commenting on such hidden aspects is always difficult, but this book is brave enough to do so.

In attempting to reveal the hidden themes, it was our intention for the book to be a resource guide, providing a theoretical link to practical observation and application. The reader will find some overlap of ideas throughout the book, though this should not stop one from dipping in and out of it.

Chapter one is a reflective discussion of the spoken and written language that health professionals use with regard to death and dying. The euphemisms and vagaries that often mask the reality, and consequently inhibit the timely delivery of appropriate palliation, are discussed. The authors explore the reluctance of some healthcare professionals to state the facts about death explicitly. This chapter challenges professionals to write down clearly what they say.

Chapter two looks at what constitutes an urgent admission into hospice care. There are different models used for admitting patients to hospice care, and this chapter reveals how some of them may be manipulated in the process. The staff working in hospices and making key policy decisions may find some of the views expressed in this chapter highly challenging. It is important to approach these views with an open mind, so that new decisions and policies are developed for the allocation of scarce resources.

Chapter three tackles the mystery of time and how best to relate to it when approaching death. Human perceptions of time are discussed from a philosophical perspective, and then related to practice. The dying patient's perception of time is also brought into focus, with the aim of helping the patient negotiate whatever time he or she has left.

Chapter four explores the benefits of 'presencing'. Although it is a complex term and difficult to define, 'presencing' is a vital part of holistic nursing and comprises such qualities as empathy, kindness and openess. It is thought to be of great therapeutic benefit to healthcare professionals and patients alike.

Chapter five examines the concept of suffering — often talked about, but seldom understood. The author offers a philosophical exploration of suffering, which is intended as both a useful reference for academic work, and a guide that is applicable to clinical practice. Although readers will have their own perception of suffering, this chapter is a basis for discussion and is designed to generate further debate.

Chapter six examines how a patient's social world can disintegrate after the diagnosis of a life-shortening illness. Ironically, this is often the time when the dying person needs to be surrounded by people — for comfort, reassurance and company. Social disintegration is characterised by the erosion of the very relationships that once used to be so central to a good quality of life.

Chapter seven explores some of the psychosocial challenges faced by dying patients and by the healthcare professionals who look after them. The author argues that psychological as well as social needs can deny the patient a good quality of life in the time they have left. Complex psychological theories are discussed in a carefully simplified way to aid greater understanding.

Chapter eight offers an insight into 'spirituality' within palliative care. The author explores different aspects of spirituality, and highlights its importance in the lives of dying patients and the need for it to be discussed openly. This chapter could be a useful reference for further academic work.

Chapter nine looks at the poor attention paid to sexuality in palliative care. In the first part, the author discusses the seeming reluctance of healthcare professionals to address the issue of sexuality. Drawing on models of grief, loss, passion and intimacy, this chapter explores how society, culture and the medical model of care have affected patients and carers alike. The second part of this chapter offers practical advice on addressing sexuality issues in the clinical setting, some of which is highly challenging and best approached with an open mind.

Chapter ten looks at the emotional demands on healthcare professionals of caring for a dying patient. The effect and hidden impact of emotional 'burn-out' is discussed with helpful suggestions on how to survive the inevitable stresses. Although it is always vital for professionals to continue helping and supporting others, the author argues, attention must also be paid to self-care — something that is often sacrificed in the carer's role.

We conclude the book by challenging readers to think explicitly about the positive aspects of dying. We believe that the unadorned knowledge that a person is dying can open doors to extra resources, high-quality care and other specialised services. The debate centres around dying being perceived as a privilege. The questions are: whose privilege and from what viewpoint?

It is our hope that you will find this book interesting and challenging. Putting it together has been exhilarating and, in the process, we have gained a great deal of insight into the hidden aspects of palliative care, as perceived by the book's expert contributors. We hope you will enjoy this book, whether you are working in clinical areas, academic circles or are still in training.

Brian Nyatanga, Maxine Astley-Pepper
February 2005

Acknowledgements

In producing a book like this, there are many demands placed upon different individuals at various levels, including time commitments, sacrifices, patience and tolerance from those around us. We are very grateful for the love and support offered by both our families whilst we were depriving them of quality time together. We thank and love you dearly.

Our fellow contributors have been enthusiastic, passionate and dedicated in helping to expose the hidden aspects in palliative care. Their individual perspectives and stories have linked together to produce this exciting book — thank you all.

Our gratitude extends to friends, colleagues and acquaintances who have helped and encouraged us during the whole process.

Last, but not least, we would like to thank our secretary, Yulander Charles, for her word-processing skills and for keeping us on track. Her wicked sense of humour was a welcome relief as we were racing against the deadline.

Thank you one and all.

Brian Nyatanga, Maxine Astley-Pepper

Dedications

For my parents, Sheila and Denis, my husband, David, and my children, Daniel and Georgina, who have never hidden their love and belief in me.

Maxine Astley-Pepper

To Cilla, Pam Lou, Nev and Lewin who have shared their love and support openly over the years.

Brian Nyatanga

1

Written words: hidden meanings

Janine Birley, Gwyneth Morgan

Introduction

Although largely hidden from the view of the rest of humanity, the provision of palliative care has become a major specialty in the field of health care. As a result of changes in treatment modalities, the need for palliation increases as palliative care continues to become known as a specialist field in its own right. This growth of a specialism that is so closely associated with taboo and voyeuristic attitudes of today's culture presents many challenges. One such challenge is how healthcare professionals write about palliative care, issues of death and dying, and document how this care is given.

In this chapter, the first in the book, we will explore how healthcare professionals' written words may mask the reality of a situation and, in doing so, restrict the boundaries of palliative care. If we start by taking a historical overview, it soon becomes apparent that there has been a number of name changes to describe the care given to dying patients: 'care of the dying', 'terminal care', 'hospice care', 'palliative care' and 'end of life care'.

The new millennium has resulted in yet another name change: 'supportive care'. These terms and phrases, used to describe the care given to the dying, may continue to be accurate descriptions in their own right, meaningful to those providing such care, but are perhaps open to misinterpretation. What appears to be missing from these written phrases is the word 'dying'. This may appease those who view death as a failure, but it may also provide healthcare professionals with a divorced perception of reality whilst caring for patients who are dying. Therefore, throughout this chapter, we will explore how we may need to keep changing the name to describe the care given to the dying. A suitable starting place is to define what the word 'dying' means.

Defining 'dying'

Palliative medicine was recognised as a specialty by the Royal College of Physicians in 1987. In 1990, the World Health Organization (WHO) provided a comprehensive definition of palliative care. Since then, there appears to have been a dissociation of palliative care from terminal care (Field, 1994). This is exemplified by Doyle *et al* (1993) whose definition of palliative care contains no explicit reference to death or dying:

> *The study and management of patients with active, progressive, far-advanced disease for whom the prognosis is limited and the focus of care is the quality of life.*

> (Doyle *et al*, 1993)

Furthermore, healthcare professionals appear no longer to use the term 'terminal care' to signify that a patient is 'dying' in everyday terminology, but use the term 'palliative care' and/or 'supportive care'. Palliative care's apparent switch of emphasis away from the care of terminally ill patients has been challenged (James and Field, 1992) in that it reframes the importance attributed to end-of-life care:

> *Palliative care shifts the focus of attention away from death and there is a real danger that by talking about and focusing upon palliation people may stop talking about and confronting the fact that the individual is going to die.*

> (Biswas, 1993)

However, by contrast, death has been shown to be a prohibited subject for discussion in our contemporary society no longer (Ariès, 1983; Walter, 1994). Far from death and dying not being discussed openly, it has been shown that it is in fact widely discussed, but once again in non-explicit terms. Phrases such as 'giving up the fight' and the 'last few days of life' are used to describe dying. A five-minute brain-storming session with colleagues produced the following list of other phrases and/or euphemisms in common usage:

- they have gone
- passed away/over
- asleep now
- moved on to better things
- pushing up the daisies
- no longer with us
- pegged it
- shook a seven and went to heaven
- gone ahead

- gone to rest
- kicked the bucket
- with their maker
- did not make it
- gone to pastures new
- no longer with us
- drifting away.

However, it is important to remember that our spoken words are not reflected in our written words, especially if we consider that even when healthcare professionals recognise the palliative care status of a patient, they have been found to censor the information they give (Fallowfield *et al*, 2002). A coping mechanism employed by healthcare professionals is the non-explicit use of terminology reflected in the written and spoken word surrounding death and dying. Hence the saying, 'we say one thing and mean another', and from reflection of our own experience, we always write another. Therefore, it is important to understand that the written words in patients' records may not reflect reality, but represent our belief in how we think healthcare professionals should write. This belief system in part comes from what we read in the professional journals and texts.

There is much written on the subject of care of the dying patient and their family. Many writers examine how the metaphor of the shield and cloak is associated with palliative care. Along with these metaphors are concepts such as holistic care, quality of life and hope. What they mean, and the context in which they are used, may differ among healthcare professionals. These words may also be used to convey a positive and knowledgeable stance, and may well have become the jargon of the professional palliative team.

It is not unusual to observe in clinical practice healthcare professionals openly discussing amongst themselves that a patient is 'dying'. However, these conversations may often go unrecorded or, if recorded, non-explicit terms are often used — ie. the words 'death' and 'dying' are rarely recorded in patients' notes. Flaming (2000) cites the following example to illustrate the consequences of using unclear terminology to clarify the status of a 'dying' patient. A palliative care nurse enquired after a patient on a ward by asking, 'is she gone?' to which the ward staff replied, 'yes'. Following this conversation, the palliative care nurse assumed wrongly that the patient had died. The patient had been transferred to another hospital and was very much alive.

This example of non-explicit terminology suggests that if we use the labels 'dying' or 'end-of-life care', these indicate to healthcare professionals that death will occur sooner rather than later. In doing so, they give healthcare professionals the authority and responsibility to provide palliative care appropriately.

However, things have apparently changed little if we consider that Kübler-Ross three decades ago in 1969 suggested that a dying person serves as a poignant reminder of our own approaching death and/or act as proof of our professional limitations. This may be another reason why we do not use explicit terms in palliative care. Parallels can be drawn here with Glaser and Strauss's (1965) research into the 'awareness of dying'. Their study described the social organisation and management of patients dying in hospitals in the San Francisco bay area, California, USA. They identified four main types of 'awareness context' in relation to the status of a 'dying' patient:

- ⌘ **Closed awareness**: identifies a context in which a patient does not realise they are 'dying'. Information is withheld from the patient. The healthcare professionals justify their actions through the perception that if the patient becomes aware they are 'dying', it would have a detrimental effect on them.
- ⌘ **Suspected awareness**: relates to the context in which a patient suspects they are 'dying' and the healthcare professionals caring for them refrain from confirming their suspicions. The patient relies on clues to translate their suspicions.
- ⌘ **Open awareness**: describes the context in which there is a willingness by healthcare professionals/parties involved to share information and concerns with the patient. The 'dying' status of the patient is discussed openly.
- ⌘ **Mutual pretence**: this context relates to the situation in which healthcare professionals and the patient are aware of the approaching death of the patient, but pretend otherwise. All parties involved go to considerable lengths to avoid the truth.

Glaser and Strauss did not recommend any one of these 'awareness contexts'. As sociologists, they provided healthcare professionals with a significant understanding of how they communicate with terminally ill patients. In addition, they observed that doctors may or may not inform other healthcare professionals that a patient is 'dying', and that they depended on cues to ascertain the status of their patient's condition.

The two main types of cues identified were that of the patient's physical condition and the 'temporal references' made either by themselves or the doctors. Physical cues were described as withdrawing treatment from a patient whereas 'temporal' cues made reference to the measurement of the disease progression against a patient's general physical condition, whereupon healthcare professionals commented that a patient was 'going fast' or 'lingering'.

Since the publication of Glaser and Strauss's study, open communication and awareness in relation to 'death' and 'dying' between healthcare professionals, patients and their carers has been recognised as an important aspect of palliative care. However, in practice, silence surrounding a person's imminent death may still exist (Buckman, 1992; Corr *et al*, 1999; Costello, 2000; Hinton, 1999). A significant point that arises from these studies is that if a patient is unaware of their imminent death in some cases, this may also result in patients' wishes not being respected. Patients being able to make end-of-life choices will be regarded by many of us as being particularly important. However, if we look at Costello's

(2000) study, this exemplifies the silence that exists today surrounding the non-communication of the 'dying' status of a patient by healthcare professionals.

Costello's research (2000) examined the strategies used to control the information given to patients about their prognosis and, in doing so, found that the medical notes revealed that all the patients in the study had a life-threatening illness, although this information had not been disclosed to them unless the patient directly requested the information from the doctors. Information about death and dying appeared to be controlled by informing the patient's relatives, but not the patient. This unwritten policy of silence was further adopted by the nursing staff who were observed to evade direct questions from the patients on their 'dying' status and this was attributed to the climate of secrecy that resulted from the strategy of silence. A salient point that arises from Costello's observations is that if healthcare professionals do not inform patients of their 'dying' status, not only can this prevent the appropriate care being given, it may also inadvertently restrict patients making choices at the end of their life.

Awareness of, and communication about, dying in our contemporary society during the last decade appears to have shifted from 'closed' towards 'open', through to 'conditional awareness' (Field and Copp, 1999). The latter refers to a tendency by healthcare professionals to control the information given to patients by withholding and softening details about a patient's impending death in order to modify the truth whilst maintaining hope (Field, 1998).

Hope and euphemism

The familiar saying within our culture 'where there's life, there's hope' demonstrates a view that hope plays an integral role in our lives. One such viewpoint is that of Timmermans (1994) who suggests that healthcare professionals try to maintain an element of hope whilst caring for the 'dying'. The positive role of hope in nursing is widely recognised (Kylmä and Vehviläinen-Julkunen, 1997), especially if we consider that a diagnosis of a life-threatening illness may present as a feeling of hopelessness for a patient. This belief may encourage healthcare professionals and relatives to conceal the truth and resort to euphemisms in the spoken word, and there is unfortunately a danger of resorting to metaphors and concepts in the written word. In his book, *Death Foretold* (1999), Christakis writes:

> *The ritualization of optimism, although useful in many respects,*
> *can also have negative effects. It may lead physicians and patients*
> *to make choices that are ultimately harmful to the patient and their*
> *families. At it starkest, too much optimism near the end of life may*

> *mean patients never see the end coming, never prepare for it, and fight vainly against it.*

Furthermore, healthcare professionals appear to change their behaviour once they have acknowledged the 'dying' status of a patient (Lawton, 2000; Seymour, 2001; Wakefield, 1999). Ethnographic studies provide an invaluable insight into this phase. One such ethnographic study was that of Lawton. In her book *The Dying Process* (2000), she describes her observations of patients' experiences of a hospice day care and in-patient unit. Lawton discusses case studies of patients approaching death being sedated and/or isolated from view by being transferred to side-rooms or having curtains placed around their beds. Lawton suggested that healthcare professionals rationalised their clinical decisions of sedation and isolation through their perception of reducing distress for the patient and that of the other patients who, due to their actions, were no longer able to view a patient's approaching death. However, an alternative view is that healthcare professionals were motivated to sedate or isolate patients to maintain the ideology of a 'good death'.

Over the past decade the 'good death' within the realms of palliative care has been depicted as that of the peaceful and dignified death of a patient which results in minimising the perceived suffering and/or distress for all those involved (Clark and Seymour, 1999; Hart *et al*, 1998; Kristjanson *et al*, 2001; Low and Payne, 1996; McNamara, 1997; Steinhauser *et al*, 2000). Or was it, simply, that Lawton observed what might be termed as imposed 'social death'? The emergence of 'social death' within our culture has been described at one level as the point at which a person dies in the social sense, leading to either a loss or change in social role and/or identity (Glaser and Strauss, 1965; Mulkay, 1993; Sudnow, 1967; Sweeting and Gilhooly, 1991).

Documenting care

Palliative care has always acknowledged the importance of a holistic approach to patient care, with spiritual care being seen as central to, and in some models the foundation of, this approach. For the patient who is facing their mortality, spiritual issues come to the fore. Indeed, the development of palliative care as a specialty has brought with it the notion that spirituality must be seen as an essential domain. Yet this aspect of care defies rational explanation or the development of 'how to' techniques (Cobb, 2002). Within the literature, there exists a multiplicity of attempts to define spirituality (Carson, 1989; Ross, 1994; Walter, 2002; Wright, 2002). Many of these definitions appear to make themselves acceptable to the secular culture in which we live. In so doing, there may be a danger of encapsulating a definition but losing the essence (Wright,

2002). In its attempt to divorce spirituality from religion, some of the literature moves spirituality into the realm of psychosocial care. The essence of spiritual care is not about doctrine or dogma but the capacity to enter the world of others and to respond with feeling. What is written is the 'politically correct' definition of spiritual, and what is documented is in essence psychosocial care, thereby hiding what is actually practiced.

The main purpose of keeping patient records is to provide a basis for planning a patient's care and treatment and an accurate, historical, complete and up-to-date account of a patient's progress and the care delivered. In doing so, in the event of a critical incident, patient records provide the information upon which a legal representation is based. Patient records come in many formats, both textual and computer-based, and in formal and informal documentation.

One of the few studies that has explicitly addressed the documentation of end-of-life care is that of Parker and Gardner (1992) who adopted a content-analysis approach to review a patient's progress notes. Their paper offers the reader a narrative account of a patient who was receiving end-of-life care. The study stemmed from Parker and Gardner's observation that although a nurse may spend a considerable length of time with a 'dying' patient, the care and conversation that take place between them often remain unrecorded. The nurses were observed to adopt medical discourse in order to document the nursing care they had given to the patient and, in addition, they recorded little in the patient records. The conversations the nurses had with the patient also went unrecorded. 'Please keep comfortable' was the commonly used terminology, which informed the healthcare professionals that the patient was 'dying'. Furthermore, Parker and Gardner (1992) report that, once the patient had died, the death was recorded in the nurse's documentation as:

Patient found at 09.15. No respirations, no palpable pulse. Husband present. Dr M and Dr S notified. Relatives notified. Seen by father GB.

The significance of this note is that the nurse did not document the patient's death explicitly, despite recording contextual events such as the priest being called and the presence of the husband. This illustrates that what happens in practice often goes unrecorded. Healthcare professionals often do not document their expertise but instead talk about it. Payne *et al*'s (2000) study showed that it is often the nurses' informal, personal records that guide the clinical care given, rather than the formal records such as the nursing and/or medical notes. The nurse's informal records are often discarded at the end of each shift and never become part of a patient's formal records. In this way, they are lost forever.

Similarly, audits of medical records indicate that events prior to the death of a patient are not accurately represented and that medical care and the dying status given to a patient is not explicitly documented (Brown, 1981; Fins *et al*, 1999). Improving palliative care for patients depends on the ability of healthcare professionals to recognise that patients are 'dying'. Explicit terminology to signify this, alongside a readiness to limit aggressive treatment, is another requisite of healthcare professionals. If we take into account that a multitude of healthcare professionals depend on annotations in patients' records to inform them of the clinical decisions and care to be given, this becomes an even greater need.

Summary

The language of palliative care is not precise: it consists of euphemisms, metaphors and jargon. Compounding this is the reluctance of healthcare professionals to use spoken or written words to define that a patient is 'dying' and to say what care is being given. Within our society is the idea that death and dying are widely discussed and documented. Closer examination may reveal that far from having an open and frank discussion, society maintains a romantic and voyeuristic approach to the hidden subject of death and regards the healthcare professional as failing when death is the outcome of disease. Similarly, much is written in the professional journals on the care of the dying, but this material too is arguably obscured by jargon and metaphor.

If healthcare professionals continue to avoid the use of explicit written words to record and define the 'dying' status of a patient, then future palliative-care provision may not be facilitated or enhanced. We must take into account the fact that other healthcare professionals rely on the written evidence held within patient records to inform them of the current situation, their practice and decision-making. Patients therefore may not receive the appropriate palliative care and may miss opportunities to improve and inform their care or their life in the short time that they have left.

References

Ariès P (1983) *The Hour of Our Death*. London: Peregrine books. 559–63
Biswas B (1993) The medicalization of dying: a nurse's view. In: Clark D (ed) *The Future of Palliative Care: Issues of Policy and Practice*. Buckingham: Open University Press. Chapter 8: 132–9
Brown MD (1981) Documenting death and dying. *Top Health Rec Manage* **1**(4): 71–83
Buckman R (1992) Basic communication skills. In: *How To Break Bad News: A Guide for Health-Care Professionals*. London: Pan Books. Chapter 3: 32–53

Carson VB (1989) (ed) *Spiritual Dimensions in Nursing Practice*. Philadelphia: WB Saunders

Cheek J, Porter S (1997) Reviewing Foucault: possibilities and problems for nursing and health care. *Nurs Inq* **4**(2): 108–19

Christakis NA (1999) *Death Foretold: Prophecy and Prognosis in Medical Care*. Chicago and London: University of Chicago Press

Clark D, Seymour J (1999) The 'good death'. In: *Reflections on Palliative Care*. Buckingham: Open University Press

Cobb M (2001) *The Dying Soul: Spiritual Care at the End of Life*. Buckingham: Open University Press

Corr CA, Doka KJ, Kastenbaum R (1999) Dying and its interpreters: a review of selected literature and some comments on the state of the field. *Omega* **39**(4): 239–59

Costello J (2000) Truth telling and the dying patient: a conspiracy of silence? *Int J Palliat Nurs* **6**(8): 398–405

Doyle D, Hanks G, MacDonald N (1993) Introduction. In: Doyle D, Hanks G, MacDonald N (eds) *Oxford Textbook of Palliative Medicine*. Oxford: Oxford University Press

Fallowfield LJ, Jenkins VA, Beveridge HA (2002) Truth may hurt but deceit hurts more: communication in palliative care. *Palliat Med* **16**: 297–303

Field D (1994) Palliative medicine and the medicalization of death. *Eur J Cancer Care (Engl)* **3**(2): 58–62

Fins JJ, Miller FG, Acres CA, Bachetta MD, Huzzard RN, Rapkin BD (1999) End-of-life decision-making in the hospital: current practice and future prospects. *J Pain Symptom Manage* **17**(1): 6–15

Flaming D (2000) Improve care and comfort: use the label 'dying'. *J Palliative Care* **16**(2): 30–6

Glaser BG, Strauss AL (1965) *Awareness of Dying*. Chicago: Aldine publishing Company

Hinton J (1999) The progress of awareness and acceptance of dying assessed in cancer patients and their caring relatives. *Palliat Med* **13**: 19–35

James N, Field D (1992) The routinization of hospice: charisma and bureaucratization. *Soc Sci Med* **34**(12): 1363–75

Kristjanson LJ, McPhee I, Pickstock S, Wilson D, Oldham L, Martin K (2001) Palliative care nurses' perceptions of good and bad deaths and expectations: a qualitative analysis. *Int J Palliat Nurs* **7**(3): 129–39

Kübler-Ross E (1969) *On Death and Dying*. New York: Macmillan. p. 9.

Kylmä, J, Vehviläinen-Julkunen K (1997) Hope in nursing research: a meta-analysis of the ontological and epistemological foundations of research on hope. *J Adv Nurs* **25**(2): 364–71

Lawton J (2000) Inpatient hospice care: the sequestration of the unbounded body and 'dirty dying'. In: *The Dying Process: Patients' Experiences of Palliative Care*. London: Routledge. Chapter 4: 122–47

Low JTS, Payne S (1996) The good and bad death perceptions of health professionals working in palliative care. *Eur J Cancer Care (Engl)* **5**(4): 237–41

Mulkay M (1993) Social death in Britain. In: Clark D (ed) *The Sociology of Death: Theory, Culture, Practice*. Oxford: Blackwell

McNamara B (1997) A good enough death? Paper presented at the Social Context of Dying, Death and Disposal Third International Conference. Cardiff: University of Wales

O'Brien T (1996) Terminal care/palliative care: what do we mean? *Palliat Care Today* 5(11): 25–6

Parker J, Gardner G (1992) The silence and the silencing of the nurse's voice: a reading of patient progress notes. *Aust J Adv Nurs* 9(2): 3–9

Payne S, Hardey M, Coleman P (2000) Interactions between nurses during handovers in elderly care. *J Adv Nurs* 32(2): 277–85

Ross L (1994) Spiritual aspects of nursing. *J Adv Nurs* 19(3): 439–47

Seymour JE (2001) Nursing care only. In: *Critical Moments Death and Dying in Intensive Care*. Buckingham: Open University Press. Chapter 7: 106–27

Steinhauser KE, Clipp EC, McNeilly M, Christakis NA, McIntyre LM, Tulsky JA (2000) In search of a good death: observations of patients, families and providers. *Ann Intern Med* 132(10): 825–32

Sudnow D (1967) *Passing On: The Social Organization of Dying*. New Jersey, Englewood Cliffe: Prentice-Hall

Sweeting HN, Gilhooly MLM (1991) Doctor, am I dead?: a review of social death in modern societies. *Omega (Westport)* 24(4): 251–69

Timmermans S (1994) Dying of awareness: the theory of awareness contexts revisited. *Soc Health Illn* 16: 322–39

Wakefield AB (1999) Changes that occur in nursing when a patient is categorized as terminally ill. *Int J Palliat Nurs* 5(4): 171–6

Walter T (2002) Spirituality in palliative care: opportunity or burden? *Palliat Med* 16: 133–9

Walter T (1994) *The Revival of Death*. London: Routledge

WHO Expert Committee (1990) Cancer pain relief and palliative care. Geneva: WHO. Technical Report Series. No 804: 11

Wright MC (2002) The essence of spiritual care: a phenomenological enquiry. *Palliat Med* 16: 125–32

www.who.int/cancer/palliative/definition/en/print.html

2

The 'hidden' aspects of urgent requests for hospice admission

Craig Gannon

Introduction

Urgent hospice admissions are a part of normal practice and their value is not customarily questioned. Indeed, a patient-centred approach supports hospice admission as soon as needed. However, there is little research to quantify or qualify the palliative care scenarios that require urgent hospice admission. This appears amiss for two reasons. First, any request for urgent admission carries a major clinical and ethical impact in determining place of care and the prioritisation of beds. Second, the required 'urgent' disruption has disadvantages, arguably mirroring the acute setting's approach more than 'traditional' hospice values.

Clearly, there is an inherent urgency to all hospice admissions — with the exception of pre-planned respite. Patients receiving specialist palliative care have 'progressive far-advanced disease and a limited prognosis' that requires 'active total care' by a specialist trained multi-professional team (Tebbit, 1999). Any patient requiring inpatient hospice care will have complex needs where time is relatively short: 'a sense of urgency is always important in symptom management' (Twycross, 1997). Admission may expedite symptom control — faster pain control has been shown for hospice inpatients (mean six hours) than patients at home (mean twenty-six hours) because of more rapid dose adjustments (Lichter, 1994).

Despite hospices' desire to meet patients' needs, immediate admission isn't always possible and requests must be prioritised. UK hospices have small bed numbers (mean 15.3 beds; mode 10 beds; range 3–63 beds) with high occupancy rates (mean 75.5%; range 48.95–99.7%) (Eve and Higginson, 2000). This leaves little flexibility for peaks in admission requests.

The shortcomings in existing knowledge leave no validated guidelines for the current prioritisation of hospice beds. Wide variations in practice exist within and between units. The prioritisation of hospice beds can be emotionally charged for hospice staff (MacDonald, 1995). Moreover, caution around urgent hospice admissions is necessary, as the distinction between palliative care emergencies from other emergencies (medical, oncological, surgical or social) is not yet described, despite being a mandatory prerequisite to appropriate triage.

Urgent hospice admissions impact on patients, carers and healthcare professionals. They can influence:

⌘ Place of care — level of intervention (eg. investigations) and possibly place of death.
⌘ Priority for admission — 'non-urgent' requests are disadvantaged.
⌘ Rigour of assessment — the urgency limits the option for further review before admission.

Importantly, urgent admissions may reflect palliative care crises best avoided. Last minute admissions can be 'inappropriate and distressing' (Higginson *et al*, 1999) and emergencies deliver negative impact on patients/families, particularly when badly managed (Kaye, 1993). Emergency hospice admissions do not fit easily within the proactive, conservative and home-focused components of palliative care philosophy.

By contrast, a questionnaire showed that general practitioners and district nurses agreed that the most important palliative care service developments were urgent hospice admissions (Barclay *et al*, 1999). And this view, along with the demand on hospice beds, is likely to increase with an ageing population and more deaths from chronic diseases (Higginson, Astin, Dolan, 1998).

The evidence base around urgent requests for hospice admission

The factors influencing the urgency of hospice admissions have not been studied directly, with any discussion requiring cautious extrapolation from parallel literature. A systematic review on urgent hospice admissions was attempted, but even after widening the search and relaxing the selection criteria, few directly relevant papers were identified. Thus it was necessary to review the literature with potential relevance. Though speculative, the research with the most predictable overlaps with urgency was sought, covering:

• place of death
• patients with 'high' palliative care needs
• emergencies and out of hours
• specific admission policies.

This literature review provided a meta-synthesis (Higginson *et al*, 2002) of the possible influences upon urgent requests for hospice admission from the sixty-one systematically identified papers (Gannon, 2003). Many limitations were identified preventing further appraisal and analysis. Besides the complexity of factors, the retrieved literature also displayed: apparent contradictions; heterogeneous designs/analyses; and numerous issues around the quality and relevance of the data. A modified best-evidence approach was used for analysis (Slavin, 1995).

A bewildering array of potential influences on urgent hospice admissions was identified. These involved the caring relatives and formal care services as much as the patient and crossed physical, social, spiritual and psychological domains (*Box 2.1*). Influences appeared as diverse as: patients' symptoms; patients' benefit from faith; denial in their carers; available support services; out of hours specialist advice; and the nature of individual staff involved in decision-making.

However, the literature did not provide a confident evidence base for practice. It remained unclear which of the identified factors were relevant to urgency, or even if they influenced hospice admission at all. Yet without better evidence, this parallel literature carries some weight.

Box 2.1: Categories of the potential influences on urgent hospice admissions

Patient's background factors:

Demographics
Personality/behaviour/choices

Patient's clinical condition:

Nature of background disease(s), including availability and suitability of active management
Nature of physical and emotional symptoms, particularly the resulting distress and dependency

Family support/informal care issues:

Availability, location and relationship
Personality/behaviour/choices
Carer's needs

Formal care, specialist and generalist:

Level of provision, nature of provision, and skills within:
  ~ local community services
  ~ non-home-based services eg. community hospitals
  ~ specialist palliative care services.

Consideration of the evidence base around urgent requests for hospice admission

Potential influences on urgency derived from determinants of place of death

Determinants of place of death will contain influences on terminal hospice admissions — constituting half of UK hospice admissions (Eve and Higginson, 2000). Urgency could feature commonly in terminal care admissions as: time is short; symptoms increase at the end of life (Fainsinger *et al*, 1991; Nauck, Klaschik, Ostgathe, 2000); crises occur requiring rapid responses (McWhinney, Bass, Orr, 1995); patients may delay admission as long as possible (Boyd, 1993); and clinical needs are sufficient to prevent a home death — the wish of most patients, though still occurring in only a minority (King *et al*, 2000).

The prominent reason for admission at the end of life appears a shortfall in health and social care in the community to meet increasing dependency (Dunphy and Amesbury, 1990; Townsend *et al*, 1990; Wall, Rodriguez, Saultz, 1993; McWhinney, Bass, Orr, 1995; Grande, Addington-Hall, Todd, 1998; Karlsen and Addington-Hall, 1998). An American study confirmed that place of death was not determined by patients' preferences or characteristics but significantly influenced by local health resource availability (Pritchard *et al*, 1998). While a review of patients' last forty-eight hours raised no specific indication for hospice admission, it implied that admission was not necessary if treatment and support were in place (Adam, 1998).

However, health and social care may not be the whole answer: a randomised controlled trial of a hospital at home service for terminal patients failed to show a significant increase in home deaths, despite increasing levels of care at home. Yet this result could be misleading: the small increase in home deaths potentially lacked significance due to high-quality standard care and low power following recruitment difficulties and high attrition (Grande *et al*, 2000). Similarly, the influence of specialist input on place of death is unclear. A review showed additional specialist palliative care at home didn't remove the need for an informal carer to achieve a home death — stressing the importance of an able carer not under strain (Grande, Addington-Hall, Todd, 1998). Also, the American SUPPORT study didn't back the assumption that the course of dying could be altered by information on prognosis, communication and pain control (Pritchard *et al*, 1998). By contrast, a recent American study in nursing homes (ie. social care in place) did show a significant reduction in hospitalisation at the end of life in residents receiving community palliative care (24%) compared with residents who did not (44%) (Miller, Gozalo, Mor, 2001). Additionally, an Israeli study showed only the degree of closeness of the key carer as significantly influencing place of death — home being more likely the closer the relationship (Loven *et al*, 1990).

Interpretation of the findings is not straightforward, typified by the influences on home deaths from patient preference and social class.

The true significance of a patient's choice of a home death is unclear. Patients may be expressing their wish for the type of death that can be managed at home, rather than an actual preferred location (Kirkham, 1994) with preferences changing when highly symptomatic (Bruera *et al*, 1990) or, as death approaches, to favour institutions (Hinton, 1994). Thus, studies may underestimate the impact of changes of mind.

Social class and other sociodemographic factors have generated conflicting results on their influence on place of death. Several studies have shown increased home deaths with increasing social class (Grande, Addington-Hall, Todd, 1998; Higginson *et al*, 1999). Others have shown no effect of social class (Hinton, 1994; Karlsen and Addington-Hall, 1998) with an American study failing to find an influence from any sociodemographic factors on hospital death rate (Pritchard *et al*, 1998). Additionally, a UK study showed a non-linear association with lowest home death rates at each end of the social class range (Sims *et al*, 1997).

It has been concluded that the determinants of place of death are a complex interplay of personal and cultural values, physical and medical factors, support network characteristics, and healthcare forces. Additional work to focus on the strain placed on the support network and consideration of more complex models of patient's pattern of deterioration and clinical need has been suggested (Tang and McCorkle, 2001).

Potential influences on urgency derived from patients admitted with high palliative care needs

Determinants of hospice admissions in general will contain factors around urgency. Intuitively, patients with high needs will be more urgent — for example, acute, severe or multiple symptoms demanding faster responses — but the literature is conflicting.

Patients with higher needs were defined in a Canadian study by need for a tertiary palliative care unit rather than a secondary hospice unit. These patients were younger, with a higher frequency and severity of many symptoms, difficult to treat pains and positive CAGE screening for alcohol excess. Significantly more common 'severe' symptoms were: pain; depression; anxiety; drowsiness; nausea; impaired well-being; and shortness of breath (Bruera *et al*, 2000). However, 'severe' inactivity and anorexia were not significantly increased and 'non-severe' symptoms were also raised. Thus, severity alone did not appear to be a reliable guide and the identified symptoms may reflect targeting of admissions as much as need.

A study of terminal hospice admissions from freestanding community teams (Dunphy and Amesbury, 1990) may also identify patients with higher needs and urgency, appearing more selected as able to overcome greater barriers to admission, as shown by lower hospice admission rates than community teams attached to inpatient units (though referral characteristics introduce potential bias). Care needs were the main influence in three-quarters, though specific symptoms were noted in the remainder — pain; dyspnoea; malaise; gastrointestinal (GI) bleeding; confusion; convulsions; dysphagia and depression — with some carrying implicit urgency.

By contrast, urgent hospice admission may not be appropriate despite rapidly progressive symptoms — the need for more active investigation and treatment has been highlighted. Many treatable causes of acute dyspnoea presenting as an emergency have been noted (Wrede-Seaman, 2001) while the need for monitoring cancer pain emergencies to exclude a variety of medical or surgical emergencies or identify the underlying cause has been described as fundamental (Haggen, Elwood, Ernst, 1997). Neither paper mentioned hospice admission within their management, leaving the importance of 'acute' symptoms on urgency unclear.

Potential influences on urgency derived from palliative care emergencies and out-of-hours issues

The assumption that urgent hospice admissions are generated by palliative care emergencies and out-of-hours crises is not well supported. If we consider 'informal reviews' and 'expert opinion', hospice admission doesn't feature in the literature on palliative care emergencies, which goes further to suggest that care should be transported to the patient in an emergency, not the other way round. This leaves no definition of palliative care emergencies requiring hospice admission (as opposed to social, medical or oncological emergencies better suited to hospital admission, or urgent palliative care scenarios that can be best managed at home).

Emergencies can be defined as 'sudden states of danger, conflict etc, requiring immediate action' or 'a medical condition (or patient) requiring immediate treatment' (Tulloch, 1997). In clinical practice, an emergency approach is required when acute events have pathology with time-limited reversibility (Falk and Fallon, 1998). Thus, a time-dependant component is required for interventions to be 'urgent' — where rapid treatment will have a better effect than delayed treatment (Kaye, 1999). To justify urgent hospice admissions, logic demands the existence of interventions that are both hospice-specific and time-dependent. Otherwise unnecessary delays could be introduced: from the time of the request to admission (if equivalent treatment could have been given at home) or inequity if the need for prompt intervention is no greater than non-urgent hospice admissions. The literature revealed few time-dependant interventions specific to the inpatient hospice setting, or the need for them, questioning the appropriateness of 'emergency' requests for hospice admission (*Box 2.2*).

Box 2.2: Areas within patients' clinical condition as potential influences on urgency of admission from review of the literature

Background disease

Diagnosis: malignant or benign and type or site of cancer — eg. haematological cancers have a high hospital death rate.

Unrelated co-morbidity: eg. visual or hearing impairment.

Severity and course of the disease: timing of presentation or duration of illness; rate of deterioration — particularly sudden and/or unpredicted changes and nearness to death; level and duration of nursing input; prior hospital stays (frequency and time as inpatient).

Reversibility: availability and suitability of active management for acute/chronic pathology.

Conditions specified as 'palliative care emergencies' or 'crises': massive/acute haemorrhage (eg. severe GI bleed or intrahepatic haemorrhage); spinal cord compression; seizures; fractures (eg. acute vertebral collapse/instability, fracture of long bones); acute respiratory distress, dyspnoea/tracheal obstruction (choking/stridor); acute anxiety/panic attack and depression/family panic; superior *vena cava* obstruction; hypercalcaemia; acute confusion/psychosis/terminal agitation; anaphylaxis; death; dying; biliary/ureteric colic; bladder spasm; escalating/intractable/severe pain; intractable/severe nausea and vomiting; sudden illness of the main carer; relief of obstructive renal failure; urinary retention; collapse; self-inflicted wound; acute bowel obstruction; increased intracranial pressure; cardiac tamponade; acute embolic phenomenon; infection/neutropenic sepsis (author's observation).

Symptom factors

Nature of physical and emotional symptoms: number/combination; acute/sudden/unexpected/familiarity with a symptom; severity; rate of increase/peaks; impact/distress incurred; duration; complexity; uncontrolled or refractory/responsiveness to initial interventions; requiring a prompt response.

Symptoms of dependency: weakness/immobility; need for physical care/generic nursing needs; safety issues; decline in ADL status (activities of daily living) — duration of dependency/functional status.

Box 2.2 continued...

Other physical symptoms specified: pain; dyspnoea; respiratory distress (stridor/choking); nausea/vomiting; seizures; (massive) haemorrhages; constipation; dysphagia; anorexia; malaise/fatigue; incontinence; mouth problems; myoclonus; weight loss; fever; insomnia; dry mouth.

Psychological symptoms specified: reduced quality of life/well-being; confusion; agitation/restlessness; anxiety/panic attacks; fear of crises as well as actual crises; depression; drowsiness.

Specific investigations/treatments required by admission: medical input/ diagnostic evaluation; starting new drug, alter existing dose (opioids reduction/ increase), make regular not PRN, change drug choice, change drug route (parenteral) or maintain prescribed medicines; analgesic/coanalgesic; (strong) opioids; NSAID; paracetamol (alone/combined); benzodiazepines/anxiolytics; corticosteroids; neuroleptics/hypnotics; oxygen; anti-emetics; syringe driver; antibiotics; subcutaneous hydration; laboratory investigations; manual evacuation; laxatives; chemotherapy; transfusions; urinary catheter; pressure sore care; suction; positioning; pressure/dressings on external bleeding; explanation/advice; immobilise fractures.

The literature on palliative care emergencies described predominantly oncological or medical emergencies requiring hospital investigation, treatment or immediate on-site interventions and not hospice admission. Although hospital admission was only occasionally specified, it was commonly implicit within the management of 'palliative care emergencies' (eg. to obtain MRIs). Moreover, the suggested interdisciplinary approach required to manage malignant spinal cord compression omitted palliative care input (Falk and Fallon, 1998). Hence most of the 'classical' emergencies in palliative care would appear more likely to be transferred out of a hospice rather than 'blue-lighted' in.

Clearly, some emergency interventions or resuscitative measures may be inappropriate when best interests are considered (Kaye, 1993; Kaye, 1999; Smith, 1994; Twycross, 1997). A conservative approach may be chosen — passing over hospital interventions for supportive care, either at home or in the hospice setting. However, this change of intent may change the urgency and even the need for admission (prompt explanation and reassurance may suffice). A personal view detailing terminal patients' 999 calls to casualty, suggested that hospital admission may not be ideal or necessary, favouring home with the right support (Donaldson, 1998). Clearly, many conditions would prove difficult to manage in the home setting without unusually high levels of support (eg. terminal agitation requiring monitoring of sedation), thereby necessitating hospice admission.

It has been suggested that 'emergencies' in palliative care can be prevented and some 'medical' emergencies are social emergencies, which may not be the responsibility of palliative care. The complex clinical and ethical components of decision-making around emergencies have been highlighted (Kaye, 1999). A hospice rapid-response service identified its key need as filling gaps in social or generic care with pressure on carers prompting referral more than patient need (King *et al*, 2000). An American study of emergency medical services suggested blue-light emergencies in palliative care are rare (less than 2% of patients), highlighting family panic as a central feature of both appropriate and inappropriate emergency calls (Rausch and Ramzy, 1991). The rate that a patient's condition changes may be relevant in precipitating emergencies: a review of palliative care emergencies at a UK general hospital displayed high self-referral, implying sudden changes requiring input before help could arrive (Munday *et al*, 2000). These may represent real emergencies or perceived emergencies as patients or carers were unprepared or unsupported.

Problems presenting out of normal working hours to emergency cover would be expected to be more urgent (as unable to wait). A recent UK review of out-of-hours palliative care services implied that there were few true crises, with out-of-hours problems reflecting deficiencies in service provision for generic support and generalist palliative care (assisted by specialist advice) without proposing a need for urgent hospice admissions (Thomas, 2001). The same author also suggested out-of-hours crises result in sub-optimal care, which in many cases could have been avoided (Thomas, 2000). This could reflect a lack of continuity of staff 'out of hours', which has been cited as a cause of crisis admissions (Baldry and Balmer, 2000).

Potential influences on urgency derived from hospice triage policies

Only one published and two unpublished policies on hospices' prioritisation of admissions were found — none was validated, merely pragmatic guides to urgency. Even with sizeable conformity, differences were manifest and despite their formalised approach they remained subjective (MacDonald, 1995; Ritzenthaler, 1998; Knight, 2001).

Ranking of admission priority followed a summed ratings from four or five domains reflecting urgency, spanning:

- high emotional symptoms
- high physical symptoms
- insufficient informal support
- insufficient formal support
- closeness to death
- time waiting
- disease progression

- children at home
- patient's location
- 'political' impact of not admitting.

Lack of clear determinants of urgent hospice admissions

The literature's lack of clear or consistent influences on hospice admission generates two competing hypotheses: first, that admission is down to chance; second, that the precipitating factors are too complex to define.

Hospice admission in England is reported as governed more by chance than by need, with present arrangements both inequitable and insupportable (Addington-Hall *et al*, 1998). Indeed, the factors determining admission could not always be identified from the notes and/or referral letters (Seamark *et al*, 1996). Similar issues have been noted in other countries. Results from an Italian study on home death rates showed irrational hospital use for terminal patients or less plausibly missing unknown determinants (Constantini *et al*, 2000). Thus the subgroup of urgent hospice admissions may be influenced mainly by chance.

Alternatively, the apparent lack of clarification can be explained by the complexity of the influences on place of care (Grande *et al*, 1998; Tang and McCorkle, 2001). The urgency to admit could result from an interaction between the patient's condition (severity and potential reversibility); the resources within their current setting (to provide comfort and appropriate investigation or treatment); and the patients' and/or carers' wishes. For example, patients in denial or carers delaying admission till 'exhaustion permitted surrender' can result in 'late admissions' (Hinton, 1994) with inherent urgency. The subsequent urgency of any situation will vary from individual to individual, according to their best interests. Thus, the observed variations in the literature could result from limitations in study design, particularly quantitative approaches:

The effect of possibly unmeasured dimensions of the assessed factors: for example, patient-centred factors — severity; impact; rate of increase; responsiveness to initial interventions and familiarity with a symptom may be critical to its urgency. A new, sudden onset and rapidly increasing pain, rather than an equally severe but well-established pain (with a known aetiology and ongoing treatment), might convey a different sense of urgency. Paradoxically, shorter durations of dependency (less than six months) carry a greater need for hospice admission (Addington-Hall *et al*, 1998); presumably, time allows organisation of care and carers to become 'accustomed' after six months.

Carer/formal care-centred factors: eg. the mind-set of carers or the philosophy of formal carers. Although an able carer may be at home, if the relationship is 'dysfunctional', the patient may be no better off for on-site care than a patient living alone.

Under-estimation of measured factors: in a study where 31.4% of admissions were bed-bound, weakness was only rated a significant symptom in 7% (Seamark *et al*, 1996). Clearly, weakness is relevant to care needs (Izquierdo-Porrera *et al*, 2001) and possibly the need for admission and its urgency.

The effect of unappreciated non-linear relationships neutralising statistical analysis or suggesting conflicting results: for example, social class where lowest home death rates occurred at each end of the social class range (Sims *et al*, 1997), or with age where more home deaths occurred at each end of the spectrum across various studies (less than forty-five years and more than eighty-five/seventy-five years).

The collective effect of numerous but individually rare symptoms or needs could be missed as determinants of urgent admissions: for example, seizures may precipitate urgent admissions, but because they are comparatively rare, they would get diluted in prevalence data by common but potentially less urgent symptoms such as dry mouth.

The effect of combinations of factors within the same domain: specific constellations of symptoms were not studied, yet may be key to the urgency of need for admission. For example, a patient with severe but controlled pain on oral analgesics beginning to vomit may appear more urgent than a patient with vomiting in isolation.

The effect of combinations of factors in different domains — less obvious combinations: dyspnoea on effort in a bed-bound patient living with carers may be less urgent than a similar level of dyspnoea in an ambulant patient living alone, and struggling to an upstairs toilet. Paradoxically, the greater symptom-load, the lesser the potential need in this example. American research on risk indicators for hospitalisation in the last year of life confirmed a complex interaction between functional status and other variables (Stearns *et al*, 1996).

The effect of combinations of factors in different domains — less obvious combinations: the different mindset of patients could alter outcomes. Generally, older females appear disadvantaged in terms of home deaths, although an Italian study showed the opposite (Constantini *et al*, 2000), suggesting sex and age were not the whole answer: cultural and family contexts needed to be considered too.

Indirect effects may lead to spurious findings: the high home death rate from heart disease (Grande *et al*, 1998) may not occur by design, but reflect sudden deaths in this group. A study unexpectedly showed that patients with better physical functioning had significantly more admissions. This was explained as an artefact from either the additional care in place for patients with lower physical functioning, or the delay between assessment and subsequent admission — allowing an 'unrealistic' caregiver to agree to home care when ADL status was good, but requiring admission later, when ADL status worsened (Reese, 2000).

Conclusions from literature

The prominent reason for urgent hospice admission in the literature appears to be social. However, complex combinations of factors impacting on the patient, carers and staff may precipitate the social crises that require admission. Changes within these multi-dimensional constellations may influence urgency more than the prevalence of individual needs or characteristics, which have been the focus of research to date. Consequently, because urgent hospice admissions are difficult to study, a broad focus that includes qualitative approaches appeared necessary for any research, with the targeting of a specific subgroup, hopefully increasing the chances of identifying relevant themes.

A study to compare urgent and non-urgent hospice admissions

Following the questions raised by the meta-synthesis of parallel literature, a study was done to quantify and qualify urgent hospice admissions (requiring same day admission) in contrast to non-urgent admissions (Gannon, 2003). The broad-based methodology consisted of:

⌘ A modified Delphi technique on sixteen hospice staff (even split; inpatient; community; nursing; and medical) — an initial panel and two rounds to attain professional consensus on urgent hospice admissions.

⌘ Review of 215 consecutive admission requests (a six-month period), comparing quantitative outcomes following urgent and non-urgent requests.

⌘ Two months of consecutive case studies (twenty-two urgent and twenty-one non-urgent), coding key admission themes into twenty identified categories alongside quantitative outcomes.

The results showed:

⌘ The Delphi study highlighted terminal care domains as most urgent to hospice staff.

⌘ The quantitative study revealed 53% of all requests were urgent. These were admitted quicker, had shorter stays, and were more likely to be admitted. Urgent requests increased through the week, with increasing success over non-urgent requests. 11% of all agreed requests remained unmet. Symptom control was more successful than terminal care. Outcomes matched urgent terminal care (93% died) more than urgent symptom control (where 71% died, mostly within two weeks, outnumbering terminal care deaths).

⌘ The qualitative study showed urgent requests, usually followed dying or acute pathology, though often these weren't clear before admission and generic nursing still seemed the main inpatient need. Clinical and ethical concerns were identified, including distress from unrealistic expectations and the risks of under- and over-medicalisation.

Conclusion

The literature review and specific study gave some insight into the complex multi-factorial elements that lead to urgent and non-urgent admission requests. This better informs the assessment of urgent clinical scenarios, to facilitate decision-making and information exchanges for patients and staff. In particular, it reaffirms the need for good continuity and the need to be wary of possible over- (and under-) medicalisation.

Urgent requests for hospice admission are important, with a high prevalence and clinically significant differences compared with non-urgent requests. Urgency of request influences; place of care; delay to admission; level of inpatient intervention; and outcome. The study also showed, despite hospice staffs' expressed views, in practice symptom control requests were strongly favoured for admission over terminal care requests.

However, the lack of differences in documented needs between urgent and non-urgent requests for hospice admission, as well as inter-professional differences in admission priorities, could question current bed allocation. Differences between the urgent and non-urgent groups in patient characteristics or specific time-limited treatments were not clear, initially questioning a specific urgent clinical need. Yet a lack of identifiable specialist needs for most admissions was seen, irrespective of reason or urgency. On reflection, the items studied were too insensitive and not sufficiently specific for the individual constellations of physical and psychosocial needs, spanning patients, carers and staff that appeared to precipitate urgent admissions. Moreover, documentation reflected biomedical convention more than holistic models hampering the research and seemingly inter-professional communication around need for admission.

Though often unacknowledged, urgent requests typically followed rapid, unexpected changes in patients' conditions, putting pressure on informal care leading to 'patient/family panic' that couldn't be addressed by available care. Psychosocial factors carried an influential but significantly underplayed role in all admissions, particularly patients' or carers' inability to cope emotionally, reflecting the gap between their expectations and their reality. The level or rate of increase in this 'inability to cope' may correspond to urgency of admission request. Attending healthcare professionals' (perceived) inability to take control and reassure might have fuelled patients' and carers' panic, reinforcing the apparent need for urgent admission. Continuity of staff may be as influential in this regard as level of palliative care knowledge or 'instant' availability of community services.

The changing mix of needs in dying patients appeared to precipitate urgent requests for admission, even though in most cases nearness to death wasn't fully appreciated. Urgency was an independent predictor of terminal admissions, with a higher sensitivity and similar positive/negative predictive values compared with specialist staffs' prediction of a terminal admission.

Urgent hospice admissions fell into five groups:

1. Patients requiring urgent admission somewhere — the hospice being the most responsive to provide the support/social care needed. Though arguably still appropriate, many appeared 'predictable' and could have been avoided had optimal care and preparation (of patients, carers and community staff) been in place.
2. Patients requiring urgent assessment/admission under a different specialty, usually oncology or medicine.
3. Patients requiring urgent input but not necessarily admission, typically generic medical or nursing care rather than specialist palliative care.
4. Patients, seemingly requiring palliative care admission, but with the same needs as non-urgent requests, appearing spuriously labelled as 'urgent'.
5. Patients requiring specific hospice inpatient interventions urgently.

Thus, it is useful to distinguish emergencies in palliative care from palliative care crises:

- ⌘ 'Emergencies' require immediate treatment that offers a better effect than delayed treatment, and is potentially life-saving (Kaye, 1999). Here, input on site is the priority, and if transfer is needed, hospital may be more appropriate than hospice admission eg. oncological emergencies.
- ⌘ 'Crises' are acute emotional upset from a variety of causes leading to 'a temporary inability to cope' (King *et al*, 2000). When occurring in the community or hospital with current resources and social expectations, hospice admission may be appropriate, even if no specific inpatient intervention is required from the hospice.

The literature agreed that palliative care crises should be minimised with appropriate planning and provision, or when unavoidable care should be transported to the patient. However, in practice, crises appeared more common and less avoidable. Regardless, a unit's percentage of requests for urgent hospice admission may be a valuable proxy measure of overall palliative care provision — aiming for lower rates of urgent requests as a correlation to better patient care.

Numerous generic concerns were identified around the patients' assessment that led to admission, highlighting a potential for subsequent over- and under-medicalisation within palliative care. Concerns included: premature requests; missed acute pathology; unrealistic expectations; inadequate decision-making; and relative inactivity in the community following the decision to admit while awaiting admission.

The impact on prioritisation of hospice beds needs further scrutiny to ensure equity. There were issues around equal access, challenges to patient autonomy, and a potential for abuse even if subconsciously. The 'gate keeper' role of deciding 'best' place of care in urgent palliative care scenarios was not well described in the literature or by the research. The 'responsible clinician' deciding a patient's 'best interests' regarding hospice admission is not clear, leaving clinical and ethical queries.

The results should strengthen current bed-prioritisation processes. They confirmed the need for thorough holistic assessments before admission, tailored treatment plans and greater awareness/openness around the true need for and potential impact of hospice admission. However, reliable evidence-based ranking of admission requests is currently not possible, and likely to remain elusive in view of the individual and esoteric nature of scenarios that lead to requests. That said, crises for any reason should be an admission priority irrespective of setting (home or hospital), while selection by brevity of life expectancy thereafter appears rational, with 'first come first served' for any remaining decisions.

A variety of recommendations have been derived from the study, attempting to increase the equity around the allocation of hospice beds, communication for patients and staff and decision-making at the end of life and aid the monitoring of hospice care. These include issues within:

⌘ Training in assessment; ethics; decision-making; and patient triage.
⌘ Changes to practice, eg. morbidity meetings and increased open communication with patients/families to foster more realistic choices and to be better prepared.
⌘ New outcome measures, eg. monitoring unmet admission requests.
⌘ Audit and future research, eg. on out-of-hours admissions.

They present resource and practice implications, and cost-effectiveness remains to be clarified. Additionally, there is a need for further study of palliative care emergencies to improve the allocation of hospice beds and decision-making at the end of life. However, the complexities uncovered predict difficulties in obtaining meaningful research designs. Specifically, the study's triangulation revealed different findings according to the method applied, undermining rather than enhancing confidence. The Delphi study highlighted terminal care issues; the six-month study, symptom control issues; and the casenote review revealed symptom control and psychosocial needs as the principal influences on urgent admissions. The overview points to psychological domains as most important.

Summary of recommendations (first of three)

Process — changes to practice:

⌘ Encouragement of a more proactive rather than reactive approach to put care in place to minimise crises/urgent hospice admissions, and address end-of life issues when patients are well enough, not delayed until inappropriate or impossible to address in crisis situations.

⌘ Increased clarity around need for admission, deciding specific interventions and perceived urgency before requesting admission — extra attention to detail within assessments, and comprehensive handing over between community and inpatient staff to ensure continuity of care. The categories for admission need to be more transparent.

⌘ The urgency and validity of psychosocial crises must be more open and accepted. Acknowledging short-term social admissions as necessary and reflecting a central area of hospice practice (contrary to established dogma).

⌘ Palliative rehabilitation needs stricter and more consistent criteria.

⌘ An extra category admission for 'assessment' (without any 'promised' expectations) when needs aren't clear.

⌘ Community staff should participate in their patients' hospice admissions.

⌘ Regular rotations of inpatient hospice nurses with community colleagues to increase common understanding.

⌘ The 'reason for admission' flowcharts may help consistency/ communication (to be tested).

⌘ Increased open communication with patients/families to foster realistic choices, and to be better prepared:

❖ Around the realities of terminal care at home and potential crises.

❖ Around admission issues to ensure informed consent, eg.

the potential for a terminal decline during a symptom control admission, or the limitations of symptom control (in particular rehabilitation in endstage disease).

❖ Complex end-of-life ethical issues need to be addressed and documented such as desire for active management (from antibiotics to cardiopulmonary resuscitation as appropriate); desired place of death; designated next of kin/ advocate (asked, not just deduced from nearest relative); wills/(enduring) power of attorney.

⌘ Increased multi-professional working between hospice staff, in particular nurses, doctors, social workers and physical therapists. Pre-admission clinics or joint home visits may aid decisions around need for admission and patient's best interests. This is particularly important when admitting for interventional procedures, difficult chronic symptoms/rehabilitation, if a lack of consensus between palliative care and primary care staff, or for terminal care. Named staff from two professional groups should make requests, avoiding uni-professional working.

⌘ Patients must have been seen within forty-eight hours for an urgent (admit within twenty-four hours) request to be valid and an immediate treatment plan must be put into place irrespective of the potential success of request in consultation with other hospice disciplines. Requests must be re-submitted if any major change occurs eg. hospital admission. Planned weekend assessments may be necessary, in addition to signing up to national and practical initiatives on out-of-hours palliative care, and setting up formal reciprocal arrangements with neighbouring hospices. Encourage submission of requests before 09.30 meeting to reduce requests bypassing the formal process.

⌘ Consider planned admissions and discharges over the weekend to reduce current inequity around day of week that a request is made.

⌘ Morbidity mortality meetings — to ensure reflective practice and audit of adverse outcomes of palliative care admissions.

⌘ Overall use of prognosis as the most rational means to prioritise admission requests. Positively discriminate at admissions meetings in favour of terminal care requests, and against non-specific symptom control requests to redress the imbalance of current unmet need, possibly increase bed turnover and maximise patients' time at home. Similarly, judge patients according to level of need not setting; blanket discrimination of home over hospital cannot be supported.

Summary of recommendations (second of three)

Outcomes — 'new' measures of palliative care provision:

⌘ Use 'the percentage of requests, requiring admission within twenty-four hours' as a measure of quality of palliative care provision (generalist and specialist) in the community, reflecting crises better avoided. Clearly, a number of crises will not be avoidable, necessitating comparison with other units to benchmark findings.

⌘ Measure time on waiting list from when agreed need until admitted (measure of distress) or if not admitted (unmet need). Unmet need should be monitored specifically, and not collated with the 'withdrawn requests' which by contrast were deemed not necessary.

⌘ Use ratio of bed occupancy against unmet (but agreed) requests. Occupancy alone is insensitive to fluctuations in demand which may necessitate a larger number of beds to ensure peaks in demand are met.

⌘ Education of hospice staff to clarify the accountabilities and responsibilities around hospice admissions and the decision-making at the end of life — in particular, assessment and ethical issues around patient triage. Highlighting the importance of the request form in guiding patients' management, and the assessment of acute reversible pathology and value of hospital management. Assessment algorithms may need to be developed. Better understanding of acute medical/oncological care is needed to appreciate the value of active as well as palliative management. Regular rotations of hospice nurses with hospital palliative care support teams may help.

⌘ Teaching/information leaflets to clarify to service users (professionals and patients) that the hospice doesn't expect to offer: a twenty-four-hour emergency admission service; longer term social care; treatment better suited to other specialties — eg. acute medical/oncological input or failed hospital discharges that may be more appropriately re-admitted to hospital.

Summary of recommendations (third of three)

Further research/audit:

⌘ Regular audit to ensure accurate and up-to-date background medical/oncological and palliative care details are available in notes. Templated notes could be used to formalise details and aid the audit process. The current weighting of managerially based documentation above clinically based details in notes around admission needs to be reviewed.

⌘ Prospective research on the admissions occurring outside the normal admissions process. To confirm if their needs are greater than the needs of patients already waiting to come in (11% of agreed requests were never admitted): admissions occurring 'nine to five' on weekdays (16% of all admissions); admissions occurring out of hours (4%).

⌘ Prospective research into the balance of increasing rapport and maintaining objectivity for single community palliative care nurse caseloads against shared caseloads.

⌘ Prospective research to clarify the true needs for admission (not the perceived needs) — eg. is provision of a safe environment with twenty-four-hour nursing the priority more than specialist palliative care interventions?

⌘ A controlled trial in patients requesting urgent hospice admission following randomisation to: admission within twenty-four hours; admission after twenty-four hours; or care elsewhere triangulated with patient, carer and staff interviews would be ideal. Alternatively, a prospective trial on a cohort of hospice patients to see which patients required urgent admission, which are non-urgent, and which could remain at home would also be informative.

⌘ Research on the rate of change of quality of life domains for patients and carers as predictors of palliative care crises and/or the terminal phase.

⌘ Pull random notes for detailed audit of quality of care by a multi-professional team.

⌘ Research analysing potential groupings of identified determinants of urgency within individuals — to reflect the multi-factorial and unique nature of admissions.

References

Adam J (1998) The last 48 hours. In: Fallon M, O'Neill B (eds). *ABC of Palliative*. Bristol: Clifford Press and *BMJ* (1997) **315**: 1600–03

Addington-Hall J, Altman D, McCarthy M (1998) Which terminally ill cancer patients receive hospice inpatient care? *Soc Sci Med* **46**(8): 1011–16

Baldry C, Balmer S (2000) An audit of out-of-hours advice services provided by hospice staff. *Int J Palliat Nurs* **6**(7): 352–6

Barclay S, Todd C, McCabe J, Hunt T (1999) Primary care group commissioning of services: the differing priorities of general practitioners and district nurses for palliative care services. *Br J Gen Pract* **49**: 181–6

Boyd KJ (1993) Short terminal admissions to a hospice. *Palliat Med* **7**: 289–94

Bruera E, Kuehn N, Emery B, Macmillan K, Hanson J (1990) Social and demographic characteristics of patients admitted to a palliative care unit. *J Palliat Care* **6**(4): 16–20

Bruera E, Neuman C, Brenneis C, Quan H (2000) Frequency of symptom distress and poor prognostic indicators in palliative cancer patients admitted to a tertiary palliative care unit, hospices, and acute care hospitals. *J Palliat Care* **16**(3): 16–21

Constantini M, Balzi D, Garronec E, Orlandini C, Parodi S, Vercelli M, Bruzzi P (2000) Geographical variations in place of death among Italian communities suggest an inappropriate hospital use in the terminal phase of cancer disease. *Public Health* **114**: 15–20

Donaldson N (1998) Terminal fears and panic. *Accid Emerg Nurs* **6**: 41–2

Dunphy KP, Amesbury BDW (1990) A comparison of hospice and home care patients: patterns of referral, patient characteristics, and predictors of place of death. *Palliat Med* **4**: 105–11

Eve A, Higginson IJ (2000) Minimum dataset activity for hospice and hospital palliative care services in the UK 1997/98. *Palliat Med* **14**: 395–404

Fainsinger R, Miller MJ, Bruera E, Hanson J, Maceachern T (1991) Symptom control during the last week of life. *J Palliat Care* **7**(1): 5–11

Falk S and Fallon M (1998) Emergencies. In: Fallon M, O'Neill B (eds). *ABC of Palliative*. Bristol: Clifford Press and *BMJ* (1997) **315**: 1525–8

Gannon C (2003) *A Comparison of Urgent and Non-Urgent Hospice Admissions*. University College Wales: MSc dissertation

Grande GE, Addington-Hall JM, Todd CJ (1998) Place of death and access to home care services: are certain patient groups at a disadvantage? *Soc Sci Med* **47**(5): 565–79

Grande GE, Todd CJ, Barclay SI, Farquhar MC (2000) A randomised controlled trial of a hospital at home service for the terminally ill. *Palliat Med* **14**(5): 375–85

Haggen NA, Elwood T, Ernst S (1997) Cancer pain emergencies: a protocol for management. *J Pain Symptom Manage* **14**(1): 45–50

Higginson IJ, Astin P, Dolan S (1998) Where do cancer patients die? Ten-year trends in the place of death of cancer patients in England. *Palliat Med* **12**: 353–63

Higginson IJ, Finlay I, Goodwin DM, Cook AM, Hood K, Edwards AGK, Douglas H, Norman CE (2002) Do hospital-based palliative care teams improve care for patients or families at the end of life? *J Pain Symptom Manage* **23**(2): 96–106

Higginson IJ, Jarman B, Astin P, Dolan S (1999) Do social factors affect where patients die: an analysis of 10 years of cancer deaths in England. *J Public Health Med* **21**(1): 22–8

Hinton J (1994) Which patients with terminal cancer are admitted from home care? *Palliat Med* **8**: 197–210

Izquierdo-Porrera AM, Trelis-Navarro J, Gomez-Batiste X (2001) Predicting place of death of elderly cancer patients followed by a palliative care unit. *J Pain Symptom Manage* **21**(6): 481–90

Karlsen S and Addington-Hall J (1998) How do cancer patients who die at home differ from those who die elsewhere? *Palliat Med* **12**: 279–86

Kaye P (1999) Emergencies. In: *Decision Making in Palliative Care*. Northampton: EPL Publications

Kaye P (1993) Emergencies in palliative medicine. In: Saunders C, Sykes N (eds). *Management of Terminal Malignant Disease*. 3rd edition. London: Edward Arnold

King G, Mackenzie J, Smith H, Clark D (2000) Dying at home: evaluation of a hospice rapid-response service. *Int J Palliat Nurs* **6**(6): 280–7

Kirkham S (1994) Admissions and discharges [editorial] *Palliat Med* **8**: 181–2

Knight A (2001) St. Christopher's Hospice admissions policy [personal communication]

Lichter I (1994) Accelerated titration of morphine for rapid relief of cancer pain. *N Z Med J* **107**(990): 488–90

Loven D, Goldberg E, Yaakov H, Baruch Klein (1990) Place of death of cancer patients in Israel: the experience of a 'home-care programme' *Palliat Med* **4**(4): 299–304

MacDonald D (1995) SARP: a value-based approach to hospice admissions triage. *Hosp J* **10**(1): 1–13

McWhinney IR, Bass MJ, Orr V (1995) Factors associated with location of death (home or hospital) of patients referred to a palliative care team. *Can Med Assoc J* **152**(3): 361–7

Miller SC, Gozalo P, Mor V (2001) Hospice enrollment and hospitalization of dying nursing home patients. *Am J Med* **111**: 38–44

Munday D, Hall L, Barnett M (2000) Symptom control following emergency admission to a district general hospital. *Palliat Med* **14**(4): 329

Nauck F, Klaschik E, Ostgathe C (2000) Symptom control during the last three days of life. *Eur J Palliat Care* **7**(3): 81–4

Pritchard RS, Fisher ES, Teno JM, Sharp SM, Reding DJ, Knaus WA, Wennberg JE, Lynn J (1998) Influence of patient preferences and local health system characteristics on the place of death. SUPPORT investigators: study to understand prognoses and preferences for risks and outcomes of treatment. *J Am Geriatr Soc* **46**: 1242–50

Rausch PG, Ramzy AI (1991) Development of a palliative care protocol for emergency medical services. *Ann Emerg Med* **20**: 1383–6

Reese DJ (2000) The role of primary caregiver denial in inpatient placement during home hospice care. *Hospice J* **15**(1): 15–33

Ritzenthaler B (1998) Admission procedure Compton Hospice Inpatient Unit [personal communication]

Seamark DA, Lawerence C, Gilbert J (1996) Characteristics of referrals to an inpatient hospice and a survey of general practitioners perceptions of palliative care. *J R Soc Med* **89**: 79–84

Sims A, Radford J, Doran K, Page H (1997) Social class variation in place of cancer death. *Palliat Med* **11**: 369–73

Slavin RE (1995) Best evidence synthesis: an intelligent alternative to meta-analysis. *J Clin Epidemiol* **48**(1): 9–18

Smith AM (1994) Emergencies in palliative care. *Ann Acad Med* **23**(2): 186–190

Stearns SC, Kovar MG, Hayes K, Koch GG (1996) Risk indicators for hospitalization in the last year of life. *Health Serv Res* **31**(1): 49–69

Tang ST, McCorkle R (2001) Determinants of place of death for terminal cancer patients. *Cancer Invest* **19**(2): 165–80

Tebbit P (1999) *Palliative Care 2000: Commissioning through Partnership*. UK: National Council for Hospice and Specialist Palliative Care Services

Thomas K (2000) Out-of-hours palliative care — bridging the gap. *Eur J Palliat Care* **7**(1): 22–5

Thomas K (2001) *Out-of-Hours Palliative Care in the Community*. Macmillan Cancer Relief: Executive Summary

Townsend J, Frank AO, Fermont D, Dyer S, Karran O, Walgrove A, Piper M (1990) Terminal cancer care and patients' preference for place of death: a prospective study. *BMJ* **301**(6749): 415–17

Tulloch S (ed) (1997) *The Oxford Dictionary and Thesaurus*. Oxford: OUP

Twycross R (1997) Therapeutic emergencies. In: *Symptom Management in Advanced Cancer*. 2nd edition. Oxford: Radcliffe Medical Press

Wall E, Rodriguez G, Saultz J (1993) A retrospective study of patient care needs on admission to an inpatient hospice facility. *J Am Board Fam Pract* **6**: 233–8

Wrede-Seaman LD (2001) Management of emergent conditions in palliative care. *Prim Care* **28**(2): 317–28

3

The essence of time in death and dying

Nic Hughes

'I feel the sense of time and that I want to cram everything into life because I don't know how long that will be.'

Corbin and Strauss (1988)

Introduction

There is a paradox in thinking of time as one of the hidden aspects of palliative care. At one level, time isn't hidden at all. There are many visible 'units of periodisation' (Fernández Arnesto, 1999) during the dying trajectory which, on the contrary, bring time into sharp focus. The first experience of symptoms; medical consultations and investigations; diagnosis and treatment; the gradual transition to a palliative and terminal phase of illness in which comfort replaces cure as the main goal — all these are, to some extent, observable events that form a linear sequence in the inexorable movement of time towards death. What may remain hidden is the tension between inner and outer measures of time: that is, inner perceptions of time that are fluid, changing and multi-directional competing with objective time, which is more fixed, regular and one-directional. The essence of time, in this context, is the way in which these inner and outer measures are balanced in each individual's perception to form a particular significance for their life as it draws to a close.

The main focus of this chapter is how we experience time and what implications that has for us as we approach our certain and more or less imminent death. Husserl (1964) warns of the complexity and the potential entanglements of trying to understand and explain the 'phenomenon of internal time-consciousness'. A comprehensive review of the nature of time is beyond the scope of the chapter, but I want to report some key concepts that underpin the ways we perceive and experience time. The chapter will, therefore, offer a conceptual exploration of time in palliative care, focusing in particular on the internal perception of time. I will identify ways in which time is seen as a problem; examine alternative conceptualisations of time; and report, from the published literature and from unpublished research data, some experiences of time at the end of life.

Two key sources provide much of the material for the chapter. Hans Meyerhoff's *Time and Literature* (1955) gives a wide-ranging and thoughtful analysis of important non-scientific ways of understanding the experience of time. Juliet Corbin and Anselm Strauss report very specific experiences of people facing the end of their lives in their study *Unending Work and Care: Managing Chronic Illness at Home* (1988). Throughout the chapter, the word 'existential' is used to refer to the experience of being human, and not to the group of philosophical doctrines collectively referred to as 'existentialism'.

The existential problem of time

Everyday language gives clues to our perception of time as problematic in our experience as individual human beings. Time is said to 'make demands' of us. Our activities are 'time-consuming'. We are constrained to use time to the best advantage, to plan and manage it, to 'keep to time' when we have a deadline of any kind. Descriptions of time are dominated by metaphors that represent it as a finite commodity, of which we may have too little or too much: we talk of losing time, of wasting time, of not having enough time; or of filling time, having time on our hands, of killing time.

Meyerhoff (1955) argues that human beings have become increasingly preoccupied with time, and see it as a burden, for three reasons. First, the decline of eternity as a felt reality in the wake of declining religious belief. Second, the increasing sense of time being discontinuous and fragmented as a result of greater precision in the quantitative measurement of time. Third, the failure of historicism as an explanatory framework for human experience (that is, the attempt to show a unified and purposeful progression in historical events). The problem of time derives from the direction of physical time towards death (and to the inevitable extinction of the self), linked with the relegation of time to the status of a commodity which attributes only instrumental, rather than intrinsic, value to the self (Meyerhoff, 1955). At one and the same time, we are faced with the inevitability of death and the task of constructing a lasting self of value to ourselves and others.

Two contemporary phenomena, one theoretical and one technological, may be seen to moderate this supposed preoccupation with time, and the feeling of time as a burden. First, the philosophical-sociological concepts of post-modernism, in which it is taken for granted that identity is self-created. This does not, in itself, reduce the magnitude of the task of constructing the self, but it may have the effect of elevating the status of time to something that is of intrinsic, rather than merely instrumental, value. Second, information technology is speeding up time while giving the impression of a greater sense of controlling time through, for example, the ability to communicate with anybody in the world at any time of the day or night through email and the internet. Other technologies, for example nano-technology, may be expanding our sense of the possibilities for humans to control aspects of human experience previously thought to be uncontrollable. Futuristic optimists predict a time when cryotechnology could even overcome the inevitability of death.

The nature of time

There is no straightforward or correct answer to the question 'what is time?' Many thinkers from many disciplines over the centuries have asked the question and have proposed different answers. There is another paradox here because intuitively we know, or we think we know, what time is because we experience it — but when we stop to consider what is the real nature of time, things get tricky. As St. Augustine put it:

> *Surely we understand it well enough when we speak of it; we*
> *understand it also when in speaking with another we hear it named.*
> *What is time then? If nobody asks me, I know, but if I were desirous*
> *to explain it to one that should ask me, plainly I know not.*
>
> *Confessions*, Book 11 Chapter 14 (cited in McGrath and
> Kelly, 1986; and Hendricks and Hendricks, 1976)

McGrath and Kelly (1986) give a detailed and structured summary of thinking about time over the centuries and across cultures. They show that each culture develops a dominant conception of time along with one or more variant conceptions. They present ideas about the nature of time in four clusters: ideas about the structure of time; the validity of different ways of measuring time; the reality of time; and the ways in which time is thought to 'flow'.

The dominant conception of time in most western cultures for the last three or four centuries has been derived from classical (that is, Newtonian) physics, in which time is seen as a singular, independent dimension that can be reliably measured (validity). It is abstract and absolute (reality). It is homogeneous but divisible, that is, consisting of successive instants (structure). The flow of time is linear but bi-directional. Variants on this paradigm (some of them in direct opposition to it) are identified in Einsteinian physics, in biological sciences, and in Eastern 'mystical' thinking. More recently, Cramer (1994) has proposed a dual structure of time that combines a cyclical, repetitive, reversible structure and an irreversible, progressive, arrow-like structure. In reality, these two structures are not distinct but overlapping and mutually influential. This is really a combination of concepts that fall within McGrath and Kelly's biological (cyclical) and Einsteinian (linear) theories.

The dominant paradigm underpins many of the ways in which we measure and think about time. The successive instants of the way time is thought to be structured lead us to mark the progress of time by clocks and calendars based on the assumption of time as an objective reality, independent of human experience. This paradigm does not fully account for the ways we experience time subjectively. Meyerhoff (1955) argues, in fact, that science in general has ignored the subjective experience of time and that this aspect is more fully accounted for by novelists and poets in the production of imaginative literature. There are two aspects of the experience of time that are unaccounted for in scientific conceptions and it is these which are the area of focus in the rest of this section. First, the unpredictable, random and unmeasurable subjective experiences of time whereby past time becomes present through memory. And second, the moral interpretations of time as good, bad or evil.

Examining Marcel Proust's novel *Remembrance of Things Past*, Meyerhoff (1955) shows an important link between time, memory and the self, which could be of vital importance in the way we see time as we approach death. In the famous episode of the 'madeleine' Proust shows that the recollection of a single event can provide the opportunity to reconstruct one's entire lifetime. This ability to reconstruct the self through remembrance of the past, through a remembrance so powerful, sharp and clear that the whole past is brought into the present, freed Proust from the fear of death, giving him a sense of connection between the beginning and end of his life. In relation to objective time, this subjective psychological experience removes one from the linear, irreversible flow of time towards death and places one in a cyclical, repetitive framework in which 'time is conquered through time' (Eliot, 1943). This reconstruction of the self is not something carried out only by poets and writers of fiction. It is an essential feature of the 'biographical work' carried out by people living with chronic illness (Corbin and Strauss, 1988).

The subjective experience of flow, structure and reality of time is captured by contemporary writer Tim Winton in this way:

> *Time doesn't click on and on at the stroke. It comes and goes in waves and folds like water; it flutters and sifts like dust, rises, billows, falls back on itself. When a wave breaks, the water is not moving. The swell has travelled great distances but only the energy is moving, not the water. Perhaps time moves through us and not us through it... the past is in us, not behind us. Things are never over.*

Winton (2000)

Another feature of time that is not reported in scientific accounts is its moral dimension. Meyerhoff reports diametrically opposite views on this, expressed by novelists Thomas Mann and Aldous Huxley. For Mann, the transitoriness of time is itself a gift:

*What I value most is transitoriness. But is not transitoriness, the
perishableness of life, something very sad? No! It is the very soul
of existence. It imparts value, dignity, interest to life. Transitoriness
creates 'time' and 'time is the essence'. Potentially, at least, time is
the supreme, the most useful gift. Time is related to — yes, identical
with — everything creative and active, every progress toward a
higher goal.*

cited by Meyerhoff (1955)

Aldous Huxley, on the other hand, writes:

*As for time, what is it... but the medium in which evil propagates
itself, the element in which evil lives and outside of which it dies?
Indeed, it's more than the element of evil, more than merely its
medium. If you carry your analysis far enough, you'll find that time
is evil.*

cited by Meyerhoff (1955)

Meyerhoff notes that a negative orientation toward time has been the most
common response across history and cultures and that in the modern world this
negative view is hardly relieved by any positive orientation. We can account for
this in two linked ways. First, the dominance of the conception of time as linear
and progressing toward death and, second, a secular world view in which belief
in eternity has declined and in which physical death coincides with death of the
self. In this situation, to find a way of arresting or reversing the irreversible flow
of time towards death becomes, according to Meyerhoff, 'the most significant
quest in human life'.

There are five possible solutions to this existential problem of time, all of
which involve chosen diversions or variations from the dominant conception.
First, according to Hendricks and Hendricks (1976), 'within certain bounds
each individual has the freedom to construct his own temporal world if he
becomes aware of the potential avenues of temporal expression', though, they
point out, this is not necessarily easier than simply accepting that time is fixed,
external and linear. They do not explain in detail what are the 'certain bounds'
(nor, indeed, how to go about the construction of one's own temporal world)
to this freedom, but we might imagine that they would include aspects of the
individual's personality, such as the extent to which new perspectives can be
envisioned and embraced; the degree of fluidity in thinking; the capacity for
change; and the perceived locus of control. The effect of constructing a personal
sense of time in this way is to re-emphasise the importance of a subjective
perspective in which the irreversibility of time becomes less significant.

Meyerhoff (1955) outlines four possible escape routes from the tyranny of
irreversibility, all of which he locates in various forms of literature and all of
which fall into Hendricks and Hendricks' category of constructing one's own
temporal world.

Religious belief in resurrection, salvation and eternal life is one route that has a long tradition. The prospect of everlasting life in the presence of a loving God has provided comfort to countless individuals throughout history, promising no end to time. Apprehension of such a life without God has, of course, created a vision of terror at the prospect of endless torment. Such beliefs have declined in western societies over the last two centuries but are still dominant in other cultures, and for certain groups and individuals within western cultures, belief in an afterlife remains a source of hope for defeating time.

Another way of coming to terms with the direction of time towards death is to deny the reality of time. If time is seen as illusory then it can have no power. This approach is characteristic of mystical experience in which all human experience is subordinated to a 'transcendent reality'. Rather than seeking to preserve self-identity through eternity, the goal is to merge individual identity with a timeless, cosmic 'self'.

Aestheticsm, or engagement with art, is said to provide liberation from the anxious awareness of death through focusing on aspects of experience that seem to be timeless, as in the example from Proust above. This is one way in which the whole self, the true self, can be experienced. It can give a sense of meaning so profound that the ultimate destination of the arrow of time loses its significance. Whether this can be prolonged beyond a few moments, however, is not established. Meyerhoff (1955) suggests that this has become one of the most significant secular responses to the challenge of death and, in this context, it is interesting that art-related activity of various kinds (eg. music, writing) has become a significant therapeutic mode in palliative care.

A final resolution, and one which brings us back to a variant conception implied in McGrath and Kelly's (1986) schema, lies in adopting the cyclical theory of time. This has several advantages. It is a neutral response to the temporal world, neither positive nor negative, avoiding the dualism of good versus evil. It fits with much of what we know about life at the species level, at the organism level, and at the daily-cycle level, as well as with much of our experience of repetitive events located as phasic or special times (birthdays, etc) or as memories that repeatedly return to consciousness. For Meyerhoff (1955), it is 'another way of envisaging a timeless dimension outside and beyond the historical march of time'. It is also a way of envisaging the perpetuation of the self, in an indirect fashion, which does not require belief in eternity. We can see our own lives as part of a cyclical framework of birth and death within our own family and society.

It is not always easy to see how these existential problems and potential solutions manifest themselves in individual thought or behaviour. One cannot imagine that they are the topic of everyday conversation. Nevertheless, as an individual faces critical life-events, they may demand a lot of attention, whether consciously or subconsciously.

Forgotten time: a case study

Another aspect of time that is potentially significant as we approach death relates to what Freud described as the timelessness of unconscious processes whereby 'the repressed remains unaltered by the passage of time' (Meyerhoff, 1955). The focus here is still on subjective, but in this case, forgotten, experiences. A short case-study will illustrate the therapeutic effects of uncovering such a repressed memory.

In an extract from an interview for the Hospice History Project (see 'Notes'), Professor Malcolm McIllmurray, a palliative care physician in the north of England, recounts his experience of enabling a woman with metastatic breast cancer talk about the pain she experienced on the death of her brother many years previously. This is rather a long extract from the interview, but I think it is worth reproducing in full. All the emphases are in the original.

If you are aware of [...] possibilities for change, then you can assist people who are finding it a very great struggle in appreciating this opportunity for themselves, because sometimes we see patients who become very withdrawn, very frightened, and where you can't seem to engage them in any kind of meaningful way because they become irritable and it's almost as though they want to dissociate themselves from what's happening; they just can't bear it, I guess. And I can understand all that. But it is, I think, an unusual, if not an abnormal response, 'cause for the most part people manage to come through that.

But when you see someone in that position, I must say, it always raises a question in my mind as to whether there's something that is deeply behind that kind of response and reaction, to do with something which may have happened a long time before, which needs to be confronted and dealt with and brought to the surface in order that they can actually set it beside them. And, even though they may not have very much longer to live, that the life they have left can be a life of great richness. And we've all seen this.

And I can remember, just as an example of what I'm trying to describe to you, perhaps rather clumsily, would be a patient who was in exactly this situation when she was admitted to the hospice. She had metastatic breast cancer and her bones were very badly affected by the disease, such that she really needed to be cared for in the bed, because the cervical spine, for example, was very weakened, and there was a concern that with movement she might actually affect the spinal chord. So, she needed to be in hospital for basic nursing care, but she was, as I've described before, very withdrawn, very difficult

[…] to please and to help, and was disassociating herself from the staff to a degree that was plainly not normal. When we went through her background with her — and I have to say this only comes after you've been able to develop some kind of a relationship and rapport with patients — what transpired was that she had a brother that she had never told us about […]. And when we were able to discuss this with her, and when she felt able to tell us about it, it became clear that this was really the source of her anguish. Because what had happened was that she and her brother had apparently been very, very close when they were growing up (this was a lady in her late sixties), when the War came her brother was called up into the Air Force […] and he would only have been, I don't know, sixteen or seventeen at the time, she was so angry about this and about being separated from her brother that she never said goodbye to him.

And when he went and was stationed somewhere in Norfolk, I think, it was on the first <u>exercise</u> that he went on, there wasn't even any glory in it, there was some horrendous accident with the plane and he was killed. And she never, ever talked of her brother again, apparently. Now the reason she was so distressed is plain and obvious, and it was because she never said goodbye, and she was never able to forgive herself for the way in which she behaved when he left. And it was only through discovering this, and then talking it through with her and allowing her to relive this experience and to talk to her brother as if he was there, so that she could actually explain to him, <u>now</u>, the way she felt at the time that this happened.

And by doing this she was transformed, you know, her attitude changed, her relationships with family improved. The final weeks of her illness were very positive, she was a very happy woman when she died. And I think she had suppressed this for her life, for the most part of her life, she had functioned perfectly normally, I mean she wasn't known to be a depressive or reclusive in any way — it was the sudden confrontation with death brought about by her illness which led to this situation. And she couldn't get out of it, she didn't, she was out of control, she couldn't handle it. Now, so I say that healthcare professionals do, I think, have an opportunity […] to facilitate what actually can happen from within each of us, if we're challenged in this way. And it's to do with acknowledging that we have value; that we each of us have some kind of self-worth; that we <u>are</u> important to the world around us; and that […] our lives do have some sense and meaning to them.

(McIllmurray, 1997)

I think this shows a very pragmatic result from tackling an existential problem.

It is a story which can inspire health care professionals with the potential scope for their skilful caring interventions.

Reported perceptions of time at the end of life: reconstructing biography

For some individuals, the work of making sense of their lives and relationships under the threat of impending death is tackled more overtly. Corbin and Strauss (1988) report the experiences of sixty, mostly elderly, couples living with chronic illness. They use the sociological concept of the 'illness trajectory', instead of the medical 'illness course', to describe and analyse the multi-faceted nature of this experience and the work involved in managing it. The illness trajectory has a number of phases (acute, comeback, stable, unstable) culminating in a downward phase that incorporates deterioration and the approach of death. There are a number of direct references to time and some underlying parallels, both of which have relevance to a consideration of time in palliative care.

Corbin and Strauss use the word 'biography' to denote some central features of the experience of living with and managing chronic illness. Biography includes biographical time, conceptions of the self and of the body. Biographical work at different parts of the illness trajectory includes 'contextualising', 'coming to terms', 'reconstructing identity' and 'reconstructing biography'. Perceptions of time are central to this process. In chronic illness, the putting together of what Corbin and Strauss call the 'biographical body conception chain' evolves over time. Faced with the prospect of imminent death from a fatal illness, as opposed to managing a chronic illness which has potentially a very long trajectory, this process may need to be compressed.

In the downward or deteriorating phase of a chronic or terminal illness, there is a timeline on which the nearness of death is placed. It is a continuum running from 'immediate' to 'never' ('never' may represent either denial, if the illness is known to be a fatal one, or an accurate perception that this particular chronic illness is not a fatal one). Corbin and Strauss suggest that 'self-location on the timeline is enormously relevant to how the ill organise their lives and how others' lives are organised with respect to them.' Such self-location is not only relevant to matters of practical organisation, but also to perceptions of the linear and irreversible direction of time towards death.

Corbin and Strauss's (1988) case studies reveal that for individuals in the advanced stage of illness, whether it is a mortal illness or not, time is constricted to the more or less immediate present. A person with Parkinson's disease who is unable to self-care except for taking his medication 'lives in a microspace within virtually a minute-to-minute or hour-to-hour time frame'. Corbin and Strauss call this 'microtime'. For a person with advanced cancer of the throat, 'death is on her mind, but not so prominently as to take precedence over the daily struggle to cope with treatment side-effects and the immediacies of day-to-day living'. For another person, a recent diagnosis of advanced breast cancer brings a 'crisis of meaning. I don't know what is really a hundred percent important to me. I feel the sense of time and that I want to cram everything into life because I don't know how long that will be'. Later in the trajectory, the immediacy of bodily demands comes into sharp focus and occupies the mind increasingly. 'I have to just do whatever I do to stay alive and use my mind to just go from day to day. It's like my mind is so engaged with day to day that I can hardly think about anything else'.

The family carers of these individuals, spouses in this case, are equally focused on the present, but for them the perception is of time stretching away rather than being constricted. 'That twenty-four-hour stuff was getting to me...'; 'It is a twenty four hour thing and you can never get away'. At this stage, the biographical review and reconstruction that is an important part of making sense of the illness has given way to sheer, concentrated hard work for all concerned. Any tensions between inner and outer measures of time become subsumed by exhaustion.

These experiences may bring about a changed perception of time that gives more emphasis to awareness of others, rather than concentration on the self. Herth (1990) observed that when terminally ill peoples' ability to perform activities of daily living became progressively impaired, as more pronounced physical changes occurred, their aims focused less on themselves and more on others and this brought a changed conception of time, to a position in which time is seen as an integral part of experience: 'There was a noted shift in their values; the future was no longer defined by time, but by family and close friends and the meaning attached to life events'.

Summary

In this chapter, I have examined the nature of time, in particular elaborating distinctions between objective time and subjective time. Thinking about time from the perspective of imaginative literature and art adds a different dimension to our scientific understanding of time.

The sense of time as linear and finite remains all-pervasive in western culture and this is perceived negatively. Against this backdrop, it is not clear how the alternative conceptualisations presented can be sustained, although some contemporary ideas and the impact of technology may offer scope for changing perceptions. In any event, for the individual in the late stages of terminal illness, progressive physical changes seem to bring changed psychological orientations towards future time. Faced with imminent death, individuals' experience of time shrinks to the immediate present: to what Corbin and Strauss (1988) call 'microtime.' Forgotten time — that is, repressed or suppressed experiences that remain unaltered by the passage of time — may be significant in affecting individuals' ability to make meaning of their life. The skilful intervention of healthcare professionals can be important in helping such individuals to resolve embedded experiences of distress.

Notes

The Hospice History Project was launched in 1995 by Professor David Clark at the University of Sheffield, UK. The project was set up to undertake and foster academic study in the history of hospices, palliative care and related fields. One aim of the project is to capture the voices and stories of the modern hospice founders through a collection of oral history interviews. Oral history is made up of spoken testimony, stories and experiences, and is a valuable way of capturing aspects of the recent past. It is enabling the project to record the life stories of a wide variety of men and women involved in the work of hospice and palliative care around the world. Since 1995, more than 200 people have been interviewed, including doctors, nurses, managers, social workers, chaplains, volunteers and many others. The interviews are done 'on the record' and will eventually be open to public access for research purposes.

Acknowledgements

I am grateful to Dr Fiona O'Neil for detailed critical comments on an early draft; Professor David Clark and Professor Malcolm McIllmurray for permission to quote at length from unpublished interview data; and to the late Kevin Kendrick for a creative and stimulating partnership when I first began to think of writing about time and palliative care.

References

Corbin J and Strauss A (1988) *Unending Work and Care: Managing Chronic Illness at Home.* San Francisco: Jossey-Bass

Cramer F (1994) Time of planets and time of life: the concept of a 'Tree of Times'. In: Coyne GV, Shmitz-Moormann K, Wasserman C (eds) *Origins, Time and Complexity*. Geneva: Labor et Fides, SA

Eliot TS (1943) 'Burnt Norton'. In: *Four Quartets*. New York: Harcourt

Fernández Arnesto F (1999) Time and history. In: Lippincott K (ed) *The Story of Time*. London: Merrell Holberton

Hendricks CD and Hendricks J (1976) Concepts of time in temporal construction among the aged, with implications for research. In: Gubrium J (ed) *Time Roles and Self in Old Age*. New York: Human Sciences Press

Herth K (1990) Fostering hope in terminally ill people. *J Adv Nurs* **15**: 1250–9

Husserl E (1964) *The Phenomenology of Internal Time-Consciousness*. Churchill: The Hague

McGrath J and Kelly J (1986) *Time and Human Interaction*. London: Guilford Press

McIllmurray M (1997) Interview with Professor David Clark for Hospice History Project, July 11, 1997. http://www.hospice-history.org.uk/

Meyerhoff H (1955) *Time in Literature*. Cambridge: CUP

Winton T (2000) Aquifer. In: Jack I (ed) *Granta 70 Summer 2000: Australia: The New New World*

4

Presencing: the unseen therapeutic relationship

Eileen Mullard

Introduction

The concept of presencing has not always been clearly articulated in healthcare literature and practice. There are several reasons for this, but one of the main ones is lack of understanding of what presencing is and how it can benefit the patient. Every healthcare professional has an effect on the experience of the patient each time he or she is in contact with him or her. Being there (one's presence) seems to be the magical but often hidden contact that will help form a therapeutic relationship. This chapter will outline a review of the literature on presencing. In relation to palliative care, two questions emerge:

- what does presencing mean?
- why do we describe presence as a hidden aspect of palliative care?

Presence defined

The *Concise Oxford Dictionary* (2001) defines presence as follows:

- ⌘ 'the state or fact of being present. A person or thing that is present but not seen.'
- ⌘ 'the impressive manner or appearance of a person. Origin from Latin, *presentia* "being at hand".'

Paterson and Zderad (1976) offer the following definition:

- ⌘ 'A mode of being available or opening a situation with the wholeness of one's unique individual being; a gift of the self which can only be given freely, invoked, or evoked.'

The holistic nursing literature provide the following account:

> *An inter-subjective encounter between a nurse and a patient
> in which the nurse encounters the patient as a unique human
> being in a unique situation and chooses to spend her/himself on
> the patient's behalf. The antecedents to presence are the nurse's
> decision to immerse her/himself in the patient's situation and the
> patient's willingness to let the nurse into that lived experience. As a
> consequence to nursing presence, both the nurse and the patient are
> changed. Both are affirmed as a professional and patient as a person
> in need.*

(Doona, Haggerty and Chase, 1997)

An example of this presence is illustrated in this excerpt from 'A patient's story':

> *On November 7, 1994, at age 40, I was diagnosed with advanced
> lung cancer. In the months that followed, I was subjected to
> chemotherapy, radiation, surgery, and news of all kinds, most of
> it bad. It has been a harrowing experience for my family and me.
> And yet, the ordeal has been punctuated by moments of exquisite
> compassion. I have been the recipient of an extraordinary array of
> human and humane responses to my plight. These acts of kindness
> — the simple touch from my caregivers — have made the unbearable
> bearable.*

(Schwartz, 1995)

Philosophical background review

The foundation and beginnings for presence is within the existential framework. Broadly, existentialism is the analysis of existence, particularly of the human being. It stresses the freedom and responsibility of the individual, regards human existence as not completely describable or understandable in idealistic or scientific terminology. Existential meaning: 'of, relating to, or affirming existence; grounded in existence or the experience of living' (Paterson and Zderad, 1976). The best-known philosophers in this area are John-Paul Sartre, Albert Camus, Martin Buber, Pierre Teilhard de Chardin, Gabriel Marcel and Karl Jaspers.

Through their writings, the concept of presence has been supported. The most well known one of these is Martin Buber, whose *I and Thou* was first published in 1923. His other great work is *Between Man and Man*, published in 1947. Presence has always been a challenging concept to understand. Yet it is a concept that only man experiences. In *I and Thou* (1923), Buber speaks of three things one receives in relation to presence: the whole fullness of mutual action; inexpressible confirmation of meaning; and the meaning of 'now', the present.

Relating the notion of I-thou to nursing, presence unfolds as the person gives himself/herself and receives back from the other. In nursing, as in other areas of healthcare, there exits this realm of nurturing. An example is when nurses provide comfort to their patients. While in the process of comforting, both the nurse and the patient experience something within themselves. This something can be described as the feeling of comfort felt between the nurse and patient. It is a quality of being that is expressed in the doing or non-doing. The nurse receives back from this I-thou (nurse-patient relationship) not only from the other person but also herself/himself in this realm of 'the between'. The nurse finds more information of himself and the other as well. An exchange of validation occurs. The 'between' is invisible yet palpable, running through nursing interactions like a stream holding the nutrients of healing and growth. When the individual is present, there is this space of momentary reflection and awareness — 'the between'. The 'between' is a dimension of being that only the two individuals can access.

It can also be described when the individual is immersed in the situation fully. The exchange between the individuals is understood. This 'between' is only seen, heard, felt when the individual is focused with the other. This 'between' is valuable as the carer (the nurse) can readily pick up patterns and information not otherwise obtainable if not fully immersed or present in the exchange.

In 1947, Buber elaborated on I-thou with his book *Between Man and Man*. In the I-thou relationship, the man is honoured; in the I-it relationship, the shared humanity is disregarded and sometimes degraded. Buber believes that we come into this concept of presence as each human becomes aware of each other's being, seeking not to objectify but to become aware of mutual humanity. This philosophical description of presence is the foundation of the concept as it is known in nursing literature today.

Nursing literature

Presence has been a part of nursing literature since 1962. The first nurse was a researcher named Madeleine Clemence Vaillot. She invited the nurses in 1966 to view the nurse-patient relationship through the philosophy of Gabriel Marcel. Marcel's philosophy invited persons to be 'presences' instead of objects to each other (Vaillot, 1966). She conveyed her strong feeling of the philosophy of Marcel and Buber, saying that the nursing practice of presence would result in the mutual growth for the nurse as well as the patient. She also described *disponibilité* as placing oneself at the disposal of the other.

In 1976, Paterson and Zderad published *Humanistic Nursing*, which was grounded in existential thinking. It encourages nurses to be there in active presence with their patients and is the essence of holistic nursing practice. Humanistic nursing is founded on a nurse's existential awareness of self and the other. Presence is also described as a relational style within nursing interactions that involves 'being with' as well as 'doing with'. 'When I reflect upon my presence, I realise that my openness to a "person-with-needs" and my availability is an "availability-in-a-helping way".' This 'availability' means not only being there at the other's disposal, but also being there with him/her and the whole of oneself (Paterson and Zderad, 1976).

Three nurses wrote of existential points of view of presence in nursing (Ferlic, 1968; Paterson and Zderad, 1976; Nelson, 1977). They wrote that presence was the nurse's being there with the patient. After these writings, nursing waited for almost ten years before presence was made evident in the literature again. In this next phase, the concept of presence and its attributes came from Gardner (1985), Marsden (1990), Mohnkern (1992) and Pettigrew (1988, 1990). The attributes described included being there, self-giving, being with, listening to and knowing the privilege in the experience, being available, giving one's self, and making a commitment.

The term 'presence' was used but its meaning was not expounded in studies facilitated by Benner (1984) and Beck (1992, 1993). A note here that in the studies done by Benner (1984), Mohnkern (1992) and Gardner (1985), they each speak of presence and speculate on its use as a nursing intervention for some nursing diagnoses. Proceeding, then, from an existential point of view, Benner in her classic work, *From Novice to Expert* (1984), describes presence as 'presencing' — one of the eight competencies within the expert nurses' helping role. These competencies were elicited from the interpretation of nurses' exemplars and observed behaviours. These exemplars included presencing stories of just being there, listening, feeling close, touching, and mindfully giving physical care.

Pettigrew (1990), an expert on pain management, described presencing as 'ministry', requiring focused attention and self-giving in the moment. The listener (nurse) feels honoured by the experience and is present in such a way that the patient finds it meaningful; the patient finds it meaningful in that they feel they are being understood.

Then, in 1991, Hines's described presence as 'a mode of being available in a situation with the wholeness of one's unique individual being; a process resulting in exchange of authentic meaningful awareness, essence linking, and thus more being (ultimate realisation of human potential)'. Hines (1992) elaborates on attributes of presence, describing them as: time with another, unconditional positive regard, being with, transactional speaking with, doing with, encounter that is valued, sustaining memory and connectedness.

Now, the attributes that Hines describes could sound, simply, like empathy. However, the dictionary definition of empathy is 'the power of entering into another's personality and imaginatively experiencing his or her experiences' (Brookes, 2003). The presence described here by Hines is clearly not imaginative, but a real phenomenon experienced by the participants.

Nursing theorist Parse (1992) describes therapeutic presence as the 'primary mode of practice in nursing'. True presence creates messages of intent. This intent can be viewed as positive, as one would not be this way if there weren't a sense of mutuality. So for the two involved in this presence, there exists this mutual awareness.

Gardener (1992) identified three dimensions of presence as nursing intervention: verbal communication of empathy, positive regard and availability for practical help. She organises 'presence' under the umbrella term 'caring'.

Doona, Chase and Haggerty (1999) wove together their separate findings from their own studies on nursing judgment. These findings showed that nursing presence co-existed with nursing judgment. Chase (1995) studied critical-care nurses, Doona (1995) studied psychiatric nurses, and Haggerty (1996) studied perinatal nurses. Many meanings emerged on the concept of 'presence'. 'Nursing presence was not problem-solving, nor was it using the nursing process as it is traditionally taught. Nursing presence was an immersion in the whole situation and seeing beyond the immediate moment of the transition point to the possibilities inherent in the situation. Because nurses were immersed in the situation, they were sensitive to the patterns that formed'.

In her earlier writings on presence, Dossey (1995) describes presence as 'the state achieved when one moves within oneself to an inner reference of stability'. Mullard (2003) concludes that presence contains these qualities of vulnerability, openness, invitation and acceptance. All these qualities create the 'magic moment' — the 'presence'.

Meanings of presence in palliative care

The busyness of the hospital ward can help the nurses, physicians and other healthcare professionals do their various tasks. However, this busyness can also prohibit those healing moments that bring about a quicker recovery for the patient. In general nursing, nurses are often so busy, and the ward so short-staffed, that they may not appreciate the 'between' of which Paterson and Zderad (1976) and Buber (1947) speak. This 'between' holds the elements: the nutrients of healing and growth. It is the space 'between' the 'being with' and 'doing to'. It is when the nurse and patient are both in mutual awareness that presence occurs.

In palliative care, however, where the focus is on quality of life, pain and symptom management, the 'between' is often felt and recognised. This perhaps results from the unique environment that the healthcare professional and patient are in, and the palliative-care philosophy. The focus is not on cure; instead, it is on quality of life, care and hope. The golden thread that unites all palliative carers with their patients is the quality of presence. In palliative care, there is the real opportunity to feel presence. The hospice philosophy allows this presence to exist because there is time for the carer to be there, to be with.

Presence is an essential thread of caring for the person who is making the transition to death. This 'between' that Paterson and Zderad (1976) write of enables and empowers the patient to let go of life. This presence also guides the family during this transitioning time, in which carers can be confused and often frightened. Being present with the carers and patient can alleviate this confusion. Presence facilitates many opportunities for healing and growth. Palliative care carers can encourage this presence and caring so as to foster a safe and healing environment. The power of true presence is evident when the patients and families say that they feel understood, heard and supported. Nurses bear witness and do not judge what is being said.

If one had a palliative care toolbox, the foundation of it would be presence. The one item that is essential is the being with, the between space, the silence and holding of the space. Doona *et al* (1999) described the coexistence of nursing judgment and presence as so closely linked that one does not occur without the other.

Raudonis (1993) did a qualitative analysis of fourteen hospice patients at a time when they felt they were being understood by nursing. Affirmation, as a value, was the core theme of these stories. Zerwekh (1995) also asked home-visiting hospice nurses about times they had made a difference. Ten expert-practice competencies evolved. One of these expert-practice competencies was connecting with the patient and family and 'being there'. Could this then be presence?

Zerwekh (1997) further revealed four ways that nurses practised 'being there'. In one of the nurse's own words:

> *First, there is being without words. The essence of me is sharing with the essence of them beyond the words. Second, is paying attention. You go in with an open mind and wait for them to tell you what is going on. Third, is being present, which is described as a focused intensity and 'working through it day by day.' Fourth, is being where they are emotionally. Be there. Meet them where they are. Just being. Accept that no-one else in our society does it. That's why it is so magical.*

Mullard (2003) met with two groups of hospice staff. The staff included the nurses, nurse managers, healthcare assistants and some of the allied healthcare staff. This hospice is based in the UK and is a freestanding inpatient hospice. What was asked of both groups was: what does the concept of presence mean to you? What is presence? Several themes emerged from this discussion:

Being there, be with patient and families, alongside of, sitting with the dying patient, just there, not being intrusive, non judgmental, one with that person, sensitive to patient and family, sense of knowing.

One group further elaborated on types of presence:

- ⌘ Physical: being there in the room, sitting with them, touch, security, trust.
- ⌘ Spiritual: being with the person, being with the feelings at present moment, talking, validation of spirit sensations, acknowledging what they are seeing and saying, reassurance, someone is there, knowing that someone cares.
- ⌘ Emotional: holding the space, giving respect, allowance of emotions for carer and caregiver, trust.
- ⌘ Environmental presence: calm, spiritual feeling.

Zerwekh (1997) and Raudonis (1993) have described the major themes of presence in palliative care. The patients viewed the presence as affirming their being and the staff described the presence as being there, being with, listening, and caring with the whole being.

Presence can be hidden in palliative care for all of what has been stated. Presence is not a term described or spoken of in the literature as frequently as, say, pain management. It is a 'way of being' while caring for your patient. It is unspoken. It is present, not being pretentious but being humble, as it goes about easing the journey of the patient and caregivers. In its own way, presence is healing not only for the patient, but also for the family and healthcare professional. Healing is:

The return of the integrity and wholeness of the natural state of an individual, the emergence of right relationship at, between and among all levels of the human being; the process of bringing together parts of oneself (physical, mental, emotional, spiritual, relational) at deeper levels of inner knowing, leading to an integration and balance, with each part having equal importance and value.

McKivergin (2000)

We all learn and grow by reflection of our lived experiences. When a person is present with the other person, the ability to express one's feelings in words with a sense of affirmation permeates the relationship.

Types of presence

There are several types of presence. McKivergin and Daubenmir (1994) did a search of all these types. It is accepted that 'being there' can take the form of both physical and psychological presence. Different types of presence have been identified in the literature by different authors. Sometimes, the literature revealed the different types or levels of presence. Their findings were based on the work of Paterson and Zderad (19976), Gardner (1985) and Savary and Berne (1988). What emerged were three forms of presence. The levels of therapeutic presence not only described the types, but also what skills were needed to practice presence (*Table 4.1*).

Table 4.1: Levels of therapeutic presence		
Level of interaction	**Types of contact**	**Skills**
Physical presence	Body to body	Seeing, examining, touching, doing, hearing, hugging
Psychological presence	Mind to mind	Assessing, communicating, active listening, writing, reflecting, counselling, attending to, caring, empathising, being non-judgmental, accepting
Therapeutic presence	Spirit to spirit Whole being to whole being Centred self to centred self	Centering, meditating, intentionality, at-one-ment, imagery, openness, intuitive knowing, communing, loving, connecting

Dossey, Keegan and Guzzetta (2000) elaborated on these levels. Nearly all of the nursing interventions can be carried out at the level of physical presence, the 'being there'. However, only when the nurse can let go of her own personal life issues and focus intently on the patient can true presence emerge. Psychological presence, the 'being with' the patient in a therapeutic environment, allows for the patient's needs for help, comfort and support to be met. This level of presence also involves a 'knowing'. It is the 'meaningful' moment. It can also provide for understanding and meaning of life and its events. Therapeutic presence can be summed up from a nurse's own words: 'The essence of me is sharing with the essence of them beyond the words' (Zerweh, 1997). At this level, the patient can access their innate healing abilities on their own. This healing experience can range from being very subtle to a major change in their life. Transcendent presence is also another name for therapeutic presence. It is a spirit-to-spirit connection and often goes beyond the interaction to a transpersonal exchange, whereby it involves not only the two people but also the surrounding environment. Jean Watson (1999), a nurse theorist, speaks of this as transcending self, time and space. It allows the patient to go beyond the here and now, transforming their reality and integrating their existence into a whole (Stanley, 2002).

Barriers to presence

As humans, we prefer to be in control. We prefer at times to be in conformity and thus avoid vulnerability. Being vulnerable is an uncomfortable state. It is far easier to remain distant than to be vulnerable. We use defense mechanisms to protect ourselves from being hurt. When we use these defense mechanisms, we 'avoid the true connection with another' (McKivergin, 2000). This can be seen as a person turning and walking away from the other. It can be viewed as being 'professional'. When we allow professionalism to permeate the situation, presence is not given a chance. Under the veil of professionalism, counselling techniques and communication skills, presence is not attainable.

Rather than fleeing from 'the not knowing what to say or do', the healing power of the nurse's vulnerability can come from the willingness to be there in the middle of helpless situations.

Barriers to presence can be intentional or unintentional. Psychological presence can be exhausting in terms of its vigilance and the personal effort required. Sometimes, it is advisable not to be 'present' where there is the chance of being depleted intellectually, emotionally or physically. In this situation, it is not a mutual but a one-way situation. This is where judgment is needed. When the individual is physically or mentally exhausted or depleted, the person is less able to be 'present' (Kahn, 1992).

Dossey (2000), Stiles (1997), Bright (1995), Bernardo (1998) and McKivergin and Daubenmire (1994) have all described various blocks or barriers to presence. McKivergin (2000) lists the following:

- busyness/task focus
- fear
- concern over what other people will think
- feelings of inadequacy ('I'm not [...] enough')
- lack of desire/intent to be present
- distractions
- need to be in control
- goal direction, responsibilities
- lack of patience
- lack of openness
- personal or physical limitations.

Stiles (1997) notes that the changing face of health care, with all its mergers and cutbacks, has produced increased workloads and stress. Staff are more focused on economic outcomes, which erodes the opportunity for the nurse to be present with the patient. Nurses often find it difficult to find the emotional energy necessary for 'presence' with their patients and with themselves.

Accessing presence means knowing the patient. Use of rotating staff and bank nursing can produce different caregivers and disruption of care. These barriers will probably mean that presence will not be accessed as easily as if there were regular staff providing everyday care.

Another barrier to presence is the increasing management focus of the nurse; thus, the healthcare assistant is given a greater opportunity to experience presence with the patients. Also, although new technology has proven to be beneficial — Bernardo (1998), for example, argues that technology gives nurses extra time to be present — it can also cause staff to focus on the technology rather than human interaction with the patient. 1

Outcomes of presence

From Pettigrew's (1988) dissertation *A Phenomenologic Study of the Nurse's Presence with Persons Experiencing Suffering* emerged ten outcomes of presence:

1. Lasting impact: recipients remembered the impact of presence in their lives long after the actual experience ended.
2. Discernible difference in a situation: recipients frequently reported that difficult circumstances were easier to endure.
3. Increased trust.
4. Increased sense of relationship and 'connectedness' with the nurse, as characterised by spiritual components.
5. Positive processing of grief: recipients of presence who had experienced the recent death of a loved one were able to perceive and interpret a healthy death experience.
6. Greater energy: after experiencing presence, recipients felt new energy — physical, emotional and spiritual — in the face of difficult circumstances.
7. Improved coping strength.
8. Decreased sense of alienation and isolation.
9. Increased sense of being heard and understood.
10. Increase in self-esteem: recipients could allow support for their own needs, felt healthy about it, and could affirm and value themselves.

These outcomes mirror the many patients' stories of their experiences of presence in the literature. Stanley (2002) writes of assumptions of presence and it is these assumptions that facilitate the outcomes. Presence is a mode of being, requiring, knowing and being comfortable with oneself. Presence requires:

- knowing the other person
- connection
- affirmation and valuing
- intuition
- empathy
- willingness to be vulnerable
- serenity and silence.

Conclusion

What unites all palliative carers is presence. Presence is being with, being there. Although one is often quiet while being there, presence is active, not passive. Presence requires an openness of participants involved, is a gift for the self and the other, and can fill the void of the present moment or future. Presence can be seen, felt and remembered. It is often assumed to exist, which is why it is said to be a hidden aspect of palliative care. It is not quantitative. Presence is the honouring of the spirit, of the suffering, of the joys of the individual.

Improving and enhancing presencing in palliative care can be done in a variety of ways. One strategy would be to introduce the concept of presence in a module for pre- and post-registration nursing students, and in all programmes for allied healthcare professionals as well as pre-medical students. The module could also explore communication techniques and the concept of self-care for healthcare professionals. Through the use of experiential learning, self-awareness exercises could be taught to the students.

Another strategy would be to introduce the concept of presence to all post-registration students in health care: nurses, GPs, consultants, physiotherapists, occupational therapists, radiographers, social workers, healthcare assistants, and so on. Self-awareness exercises could also be introduced into communication workshops. By these measures, presence will no longer be a hidden aspect of palliative care but very much an integral component.

The following quotation provides a poignant account of presencing and is a fitting end to the chapter:

I am still bound upon Lear's heel of fire, but the love and devotion of my family and friends, and the deep caring and engagement of my caregivers, have been a tonic for my soul and have helped to take some of the sting from my scalding tears.

(Kenneth and Schwartz, 1995)

References

Beck ST (1992) Caring among nursing students. *Nurse Educ* **17**: 22–7

Beck ST (1993) Caring relationships between nursing students and their patients. *Nurse Educ* **18**: 28–32

Benner B (1984) *From Novice to Expert: Excellence and Power in Clinical Nursing Practice*. Menlo Park, CA: Addison-Wesley

Bernardo A (1998) Technology and true presence in nursing. *Holist Nurs Pract* **12**(4): 40–9

Bright MA (1995) Centering: the path to healing presence. *Altern Health Pract* **1**(3): 191–4

Brookes I (ed) (2003) *The Chambers Dictionary*. Edinburgh: Chambers Harrap

Buber M (1958) *I and Thou*. Edinburgh: T&T Clark Ltd

Buber M (1947) *Between Man and Man*. London: Collins Clear-Type Press

Chase SK (1995) The social context of critical care clinical judgment. *Heart Lung* **24**: 154–62

Doona ME (1995) Nurses' judgment as they care for persons who exhibit impaired judgment. *J Prof Nurs* **12**: 98–109

Doona ME, Haggerty LA, Chase SK (1997) Nursing presence: an existential exploration of the concept. *Sch Inq Nurs Pract* **11**: 3–16

Doona ME, Haggerty LA, Chase SK (1999) Nursing presence: as real as a milky way bar. *J Holist Nurs* **17**(1): 54–70

Dossey BM (1995) Nurse as healer. In: Dossey BM, Keegan L, Guzzetta CE, Kolkmeier LG (eds) *Holistic Nursing: A Handbook for Practice*. 2nd ed. Gaithersburg, MD: Aspen

Ferlic A (1968) Existential approach in nursing. *Nurs Outlook* **16**: 30–3

Gardner D (1985) Presence. In: Bulechek G, McCloskey J (eds) *Nursing Interventions: Essential Nursing Treatments*. Philadelphia: PA Saunders

Haggerty LA (1996) Assessment parameters and indicators in expert intrapartal nursing decisions. *J Gynecol Neonat Nurs* **25**: 491–9

Hines D (1991) The Development of the Measurement Presence Scale: PhD dissertation. Texas Women's University, USA

Hines D (1992) Presence: discovering the artistry in relating. *J Holist Nurs* **10**: 294–305

Kahn WA (1992) To be fully there: psychological presence at work. *Hum Relat* **45**: 321–49

Marsden C (1990) Real presence. *Heart Lung* **19**: 540–1

McKivergin MJ, Daubenmire MJ (1994) The healing process of presence. *J Holist Nurs* 12: 65–81

McKivergin M (2000) The nurse as an instrument of healing. In: Dossey BM, Keegan L, Guzzetta CE (eds) *Holistic Nursing: A Handbook for Practice*. 3rd ed. Gaithersburg, MD: Aspen

Mohnkern SM (1992) Presence in Nursing: its Antecedents, Defining Attributes and Consequences: unpublished dissertation. University of Texas, USA

Mullard E (2003) Unpublished Findings of Hospice Focus Group. University of Leeds, UK

Nelson MJ (1977) Existentialism in Nursing: A Philosophical Investigation of Encounter: unpublished dissertation. Columbia University, USA

Parse RR (1992) Human becoming: Parse's theory of nursing. *Nurs Sci Q* **5**: 35–42

Paterson JG, Zderdad LT (1976) *Humanistic Nursing*. Wiley: New York

Pearsall J (ed) (2001) *Concise Oxford Dictionary*. Oxford: OUP

Pettigrew JM (1988) A phenomenological study of the nurse's presence with persons experiencing suffering: unpublished dissertation. Texas Woman's University, USA

Pettigrew J (1990) Intensive nursing care: the ministry of presence. *Crit Care Nurs Clin North Am* **2**: 503–8

Raudonis BM (1993) The meaning and impact of empathic relationships in hospice nursing. *Cancer Nurs* **16**: 304–9

Savay L, Berne P (1988) *Kything: the Art of Spiritual Presence*. New York: Paulist

Schwartz KB (1995) A patient's story. *Boston Globe Magazine*: 1–8

Stanley K (2002) The healing power of presence: respite from the fear of abandonment. *Oncol Nurs Forum* **29**(6): 935–40

Stiles K (1997) Being there: the healing power of presence. *Alt Complement Therapies* **April**: 133–9

Vaillot MC (1966) Existentialism: a philosophy of commitment. *Am J Nurs* **66**: 500–05

Watson J (1999) *Nursing: Human Science and Human Care*. Sudbury, MA: Jones and Bartlett

Zerweh JV (1995) A family caregiving model for hospice nursing. *Hosp J* **10**: 27–44

Zerweh JV (1997) The practice of presencing. *Semin Oncol Nurs* **13**(4): 260–2

5

The concept of suffering: a hidden phenomenon

Brian Nyatanga

Introduction

The concept of suffering appears to have an intuitive clarity of meaning and yet the numerous definitions (eg. Frankl, 1962; Cassell, 1992; Rodgers and Cowles, 1997; Edwards, 1998; Van Hooft, 1998) suggest its essence is much more elusive. At the intuitive level, it can be argued that suffering results when individuals find themselves in a situation in which they would prefer not to be — a negative experience that demands endurance. Whilst suffering may be largely a personal issue, there has to be a general understanding of what it means to suffer. This chapter will elucidate some key aspects of suffering.

Attempted definitions of this elusive concept suggest it to be any feeling of distress, discomfort or what Dan (2001) calls 'negative utilitarianism' (NU). Dan (2001) uses this term to denote the least amount of suffering a person can have and still recognise it as suffering. NU makes sense because it acknowledges the subjectivity of both the experiences of suffering and its interpretation. The opposite of this approach would be the objective dimension of suffering where a third person makes an interpretation of someone else's suffering experience. While this may appear to be acceptable, it may ignore individual differences such as previous experiences, culture and level of awareness which give meaning to the experience for the sufferer.

It is tempting to argue that the concept of suffering does not exist at all. However, this would be a more difficult position to sustain since people already talk about it. It is therefore more plausible to try to understand this hidden phenomenon, its nature and origin as well as the relationship it has (or not) with pain in both good health and ill health.

The need for a general understanding of suffering is in itself an acknowledgement that there are various ways of viewing the concept. Suffering can be understood from many perspectives, including its origins: philosophical, medical, nursing and historical. This chapter will explore in detail these views of suffering, while focusing on the practice of palliative care.

One of the arguments will focus on the fact that death and dying (key characteristics of palliative care) have a link with suffering. This raises questions of how nursing assesses suffering, what is actually assessed, and the types of intervention deemed effective to alleviate that suffering. It can also be argued that to asses for something, one needs to have an understanding of the nature of what is to be assessed, and the nursing perspective will be sought.

This chapter begins therefore with an exploration of the biblical origins of suffering, before exploring the philosophical and medical perspectives. Philosophical dimensions of suffering begin with an understanding of what it is to be a person, and where within that person suffering occurs or is captured. The discussion about the person centres on the body-mind relationship, and whether the person can be seen in such dualistic terms. The medical understanding of suffering is attempted through critical analysis of the work of Cassell (1992) and Van Hooft (1998). The limitations or vulnerability of each piece of work is highlighted, and the consequences to clinical practice drawn into focus.

Whilst the relief of suffering is undoubtedly a prerequisite for healthcare professionals working with the dying, there is a lack of agreement on how nursing views suffering. In the absence of clear evidence on a view of suffering, nursing has claimed to relieve suffering and this raises questions about what is being relieved, or whose suffering this may be, if suffering is not clearly understood. Many commentators, including Edwards (2001), have advanced similar arguments for understanding suffering, which are helpful in presenting the following argument.

One origin of suffering

In a biblical sense, suffering is a consequence of human disobedience to God. The Bible claims that Adam and Eve sinned when they both ate the forbidden fruit and as a result were expelled from the Garden of Eden (Genesis 2: 3). It is claimed that Adam and Eve had an idyllic life before this temptation and that their expulsion signalled the start of suffering for humankind. Punishment for Eve (representing the female species) was to experience pain in pregnancy and in giving birth, while Adam (representing the male species) had to endure hard work and sweat for the rest of his life to produce food in order to live.

However, in today's world, it is not convincing to suggest that men always undergo such hardship in order to survive. Bill Gates, the founder of Microsoft, for example, could hardly be described as suffering because he works so hard for his wealth and fortune. As for women, not all suffer while giving birth because of advances in medical science such as pain relief, epidural analgesia and, increasingly, caesarean births. Some women, for a variety of reasons, never have children and so are spared the 'suffering' of labour altogether.

Using Adam and Eve's punishment, it can be argued that suffering was synonymous with sin and therefore equated to hardship. This view seems to have influenced the negative associations of the term 'suffering'. For example, any typical English dictionary's definition of suffering tends to emphasise such factors as endurance of pain, grief, injury, loss and so on.

Is it possible or conceivable that suffering could occur in a positive way? Could suffering result in hope? For example, natural child birth is often characterised by pain, but some women might consider this a positive experience in that a brand-new human life is at the end of it. The proponents of suffering as a negative experience would reject this, of course, on the grounds that if the sufferer 'enjoyed' the experience, then surely it is not suffering, but something else.

It is important to highlight that the careless use of the term 'suffering' often renders it meaningless. Suffering is used with reference to distress, anguish, pain, acute and chronic discomfort, disadvantage, submission and tolerance. From this list, it can be seen that suffering applies to the physical as well as to the mental aspects of the person. But can both the physical and mental aspects of suffering be captured? It does not seem possible to capture physical suffering without the mental component. In other words, it is logical to reject any physical suffering unless it can be interpreted at a mental level. For example, a painful leg does not suffer — it is the person with that leg who suffers. It follows from this that mindless bodies would not be capable of experiencing suffering.

This implication has serious consequences for those patients who are unconscious or in a persistent vegetative state (PVS). It is often in these circumstances that healthcare professionals use the third-person perspective (objective) to make a judgement on another's (the patient's) behalf. Whilst this method is not perfect, it is the most plausible given the circumstances, and suggests that healthcare professionals do not support the precept that mindless bodies are incapable of suffering.

Before we look at whether a distinction between pain and suffering exists, it is important to consider the problems with definitions of suffering. After this, we will turn our attention to the medical perspectives of suffering offered by Cassell and Van Hooft.

The difficulty of defining suffering

The attempts made so far to define suffering have failed to be conclusive because of the contexts and values people ascribe to suffering. From a medical perspective, suffering is often defined from the third-person perspective, relying heavily on the skills of another person to accurately interpret the behaviours (eg. facial expressions) observed and reducing these to pain, distress or suffering. The defenders of this approach believe it is the best way to prescribe treatments and interventions necessary to alleviate suffering. This kind of intervention is based on an inherent assumption that the cause and nature of the suffering is well-understood and can therefore be treated successfully. Here, perhaps, it is the person treating and not necessarily the one being treated, who defines outcomes and/or success.

This approach is questionable in that the perspective of the 'treater' and that of the 'sufferer' may not always match. For example, the same facial expression may have different cultural connotations for the sufferer than for the observer. And even if the observer and sufferer are from the same cultural background, it does not necessarily guarantee congruence in the interpretation of the facial expression. Regardless of these differences, it is still the third-person perspective that creates the problem of understanding suffering. Suffering is also relative, in that what may be suffering to one person can be pleasurable to another. The same facial expression, for example, could result from distress or from pleasure.

To capture the essence of suffering, the first-person (subjective) perspective seems more plausible than the third person if we are to understand the exact nature of the suffering. This is particularly relevant if successful interventions are to be achieved for the patient or the person who is suffering.

Can we rely on science to help?

Most things can be understood through the rigour of science, so it is worthwhile spending some time examining whether science can help in capturing the concept of suffering. Science has long been regarded as the source of true knowledge, maybe because of the reliability of facts systematically gathered to arrive at this truth. In other words, science takes the objective dimension to arrive at an outcome, truth or knowledge. This objective dimension demands that the facts gathered should be open to verification by another person. The emphasis of science is on rationality. It is important to analyse the methods used in gathering data, its analysis, and whether outcomes or results can also be applied to other similar subjects. In scientific terms, it is the generalisability of the results that makes the science credible. However, it needs to be discussed whether science and its reductive methods can capture the concept of suffering.

The first point to establish is whether suffering is a credible object of scientific inquiry, in which the data must be readily studied from a third-person perspective. According to Cassell (1991), 'suffering is ultimately a personal matter — something whose presence and extent can only be known to the sufferer.'

Cassell's statement suggests that suffering can only be determined and accurately understood from a first-person perspective. In that case, it is arguable that such data is therefore not open to verification from the third-person perspective because of its subjective nature and creates problems of credibility with generalisation beyond the sufferer. If we accept Cassell's view, then suffering cannot be a suitable subject for scientific investigation.

The second point is that suffering is neither tangible nor physical in nature, but an abstraction. It can be argued that suffering is often determined by the significance it has for the sufferer, making it difficult to measure objectively. Frankl (1962) claims that man is not bothered by suffering alone, man is bothered by suffering without a meaning. To ascribe a meaning to something involves cognitive and affective processes, which might draw on values, beliefs, cultural persuasion and past experiences.

The close alignment that medicine holds or strives for with science may suggest that it too, like science, cannot accurately capture the concept of suffering objectively. This, however creates a dilemma for medicine whose goals, according to Cassell, include the relief of suffering. From the medical perspective, the identification of the problem (diagnosis) is a pre-requisite to finding the right course of action (treatment). Therefore, it is possible that the suffering medicine purports to relieve may be very different from that being experienced by the patient. Similarly, the patient may view his suffering as an excruciating immediacy, while the physician may want to delay intervention until after forty-eight hours of patient rest and the results of tests are known. Such discrepancies tend to be experienced too often, causing unnecessary distress for the patient and relatives.

The foregoing arguments tend to be sympathetic to the subjective dimensions of determining and capturing suffering. However, let us now turn to pain and suffering and discuss whether they are are different or the same.

Is pain distinct from suffering?

Since, historically, pain and suffering are closely associated, it is crucially important to discuss whether there is a distinction between them. There are two main schools of thought on this, one which sees pain and suffering as distinct and the other which sees no distinction. The proponents of 'no distinction' argue that trying to 'create' a distinction is like debating the body-mind duality of Descartes, which is up to now inconclusive. They also argue that pain is one of several forms of suffering. For example, Van Hooft (1998) argues that pain and malady (disease and other conditions) are forms of suffering.

Conversely, proponents of 'distinction' argue that one can experience pain without suffering and/or suffer without experiencing pain. It is not clear how one can suffer without experiencing pain, and how this suffering is induced. One logical explanation is to view pain in this instance as being restricted to physical experience. According to Forbes and Faull (1998), pain is more than just physical; it also occurs as a psychological, emotional and spiritual experience. They claim that, 'pain is essentially subjective as it is identified and quantified as what the patient says hurts, and is individual to the person experiencing it'. Forbes and Faull, Twycross (1994) and Nyatanga (2001) acknowledge the existence of the 'total' pain, which includes the psychological, emotional, social and spiritual experiences. These different types of pain are interpreted at the mental level of a person.

For one to suffer without pain would suggest that pain is restricted only to physical (ie. physiological) experience. Such a view brings with it the criticism that viewing pain in this way is too limited. It is more logical to subscribe to the hypothesis that suffering is more fundamental than pain (Van Hooft, 1998). A more plausible hypothesis supports this view, but goes on to argue that pain is a pre-requisite for suffering. In this hypothesis, pain is viewed as more than physical and suffering is experienced at a mental level. This is a rejection of the view that suffering can occur without pain, unless the pain is physical only.

A medical perspective on suffering

Cassell proffers a definition of suffering as 'the state of severe distress associated with events that threaten the intactness of person' (Cassell, 1991) and suggests that whatever drastically threatens a part, thereby threatens the whole. He says what constitutes a person without attempting a definition. The constituents include: character, personality, a concept of future, a lived past, a body and a relationship with the body, an unconscious and a private life. It is clear from this list that Cassell is making a distinction between persons and bodies or objects. To be a person, one has to be able to experience events and be capable of an interaction.

Cassell's concept of suffering relies heavily on the subjective dimension or the first-person perspective (Cassell, 1992). He argues that there is a distinction between pain and suffering, giving the example that, exposed to the same kind of pain, some people will suffer while others will not. This shows that whilst pain is not the same as suffering, it may in some cases lead to suffering.

At the same time, however, Cassell states that suffering may be present in the absence of pain: 'suffering may be present in the absence of any symptoms, as in the suffering caused by helplessly watching the terrible pain of a loved one'. This is plausible if pain only manifests itself physically, and suffering is being judged from the third-person perspective. As I argued earlier, pain is more than just physical and for suffering to occur, therefore, there must be an underlying cause. In Cassell's example, symptoms can be defined as the observed behaviour or measurable manifestation of some internal process taking place within the person watching a loved one in pain. There seems to be an apparent disregard of the significance of any symptoms that may not be observable but nevertheless experienced by that person. It is true, however, to suggest that this internal process is provoked by an event — in this case, watching a loved one in terrible pain. Arguably, watching someone's agony is processed within the mind, often resulting in the relative (the one watching) experiencing some distress. It needs to be clearly stated that this distress is not the same as the pain experienced by the loved one, since it is not possible for one person to experience another person's pain. The point is that this distress is not physical, but may be psychological or emotional pain, depending on the part of the mind it affects. In a loving relationship, it is assumed that an affectionate bond exists between partners and pain experienced by one and witnessed by the other affects this bond. As a consequence, the other person experiences distress. Cassell refers to this distress as suffering and therefore it occurs without pain. The earlier example shows the limitations of such a claim. It is also argued here that such suffering is a result of either psychological or emotional pain experienced by the person watching. This view can be challenged, since not everyone who watches someone in pain ends up experiencing pain themselves. The difference lies in the presence or not of the affectionate bonds between any two people.

Cassell also raises another point that helps us to know that suffering is a characteristic of persons rather than bodies. According to Cassell, without a concept of the future, suffering cannot occur. This point is useful in its categorical stance that suffering occurs at the mental level in persons and not in bodies or objects. Persons must have the mental capability to capture concepts such as the future. From this, it is clear that plants, rocks and animals would not experience suffering.

With animals, however, there may be a language barrier, which makes this debatable. From earlier experience of working with animals on a farm, cows in particular seemed to behave in certain ways each time one of their calves died. This behaviour of mooing loudly, and pacing around the dead body, was suggestive of distress, or mourning the dead (in analogous human terms). Obviously, the language barrier with the cows makes this an educated guess. It is not clear though whether animals have their own concept of a future, loss, or such similar other outlook on life.

According to Cassell, the concepts of past and present are also essential constituents for suffering. Without these, the future would be meaningless. There are far-reaching clinical implications of this view, since it excludes some patients from being able to experience suffering (eg. neonates and those with certain mental diseases). Neonates, for example, have no concept of a future until they have developed to a stage where they can fully appreciate themselves, their past, and the present. Those with Alzheimer's disease do not always remember things, particularly the immediate present. So are these groups excluded from suffering? It would be false to exclude them from suffering on the basis that they are not able to articulate their own concept of a future. Surely those with mental diseases must have had a concept before their illness, and it is absurd for the carers and/or family not to carry that forward on their behalf. Whilst it is obvious that, during such illness, we can not understand their concept of a future, this does not necessarily mean it is non-existent.

Cassell suggests that we are made of different entities (all of a piece). He writes, 'reflecting on the suffering should make it possible to see that there is nothing about the body that is not also psychological and social, nothing social that is not physical and psychological, and nothing psychological that is not physical and social' (1992). This is interesting in that, here, Cassell acknowledges the psycho-social dimension of a person, but does not do so in relation to pain, arguing that only the physical dimension is pertinent to suffering.

Cassell makes the point that most suffering may be silent and unobservable and that it may even be unknown to the sufferer. This raises two important questions. First, is it possible for someone to suffer without knowing it? Second, whose perspective is acceptable to determine what is suffering? Let us consider the following example in an attempt to answer these two questions.

A young girl growing up under a repressive sociopolitical regime is physically assaulted and deprived of education. For her, having known no other experience, this abuse is normal. It can be argued, from a third person's perspective, that she is suffering, but without being aware of it. It also follows that the person making the judgement knows of other, different, sociopolitical settings. Suffering for this girl may coincide with the moment she becomes aware of the abnormality of her earlier life experiences. Before this awareness, it is correct to refer to her experience as painful, distressing or in similar other terms, but consequently the effect of such suffering may be disruptive of her future life.

Another medical view of suffering

The view of suffering posited by Van Hooft offers a different perspective from that of Cassell's. He takes the view that suffering is best captured from the third-person (objective) perspective (Van Hooft, 1998). In his discussion, Van Hooft avoids making any distinction between pain and suffering, seeing pain as one of the many possible forms of suffering. He also states that he 'understands pain as a physical sensation'. This view of understanding pain and restricting it to physical experience seems dangerously limited, since pain is now viewed more broadly than physiological sensations to include psycho-social, spiritual and emotional aspects (Forbes and Faull, 1998).

When compared with pain, Van Hooft's (1998) hypothesis is that suffering is the more fundamental concept. He also argues that being sick and malady are both forms of suffering. When taken in a medical context, as it should be, this view leads to the determination of the goals of medicine, which include the relief of suffering. It is worth emphasising that Van Hooft's thinking is influenced by Aristotelian philosophy, which identifies a human being as having four distinct parts:

⌘ The vegetative — a person's biological functioning.
⌘ The appetitive — a person's desiring and emotional functioning.
⌘ The deliberative — a person's rational and practical dimension.
⌘ The contemplative — a person's sense of the meaningfulness of his or her existence.

These four aspects are separated here only for purposes of discussion; otherwise, they are intertwined with each other. Van Hooft gives an example of a glass globe, which changes colours each time a different colour bulb is introduced. The metaphor demonstrates how suffering at one level will pervade the other three. The combination of these four results in our wholeness and integration as a person. Van Hooft posits his first claim that suffering should be understood as the frustration of the tendency towards fulfilment of these four aspects. For example, malady (diseases or conditions that threaten health) causes suffering at the vegetative level of the person, interfering with the biological functioning. Van Hooft goes on to state that, 'persons can be said to be suffering in this physical way even when they are not aware of it. It follows that suffering is not a function of consciousness, or mental epiphenomenon which supervenes on malady'. Two philosophical points are thus being made:

i). Suffering can occur without the sufferer's awareness (or knowledge) of it.
ii). One does not need mental capability to experience suffering.

It follows from these points that neonates, those in a persistent vegetative state or those with Alzheimer's disease can all suffer. It is plausible therefore to argue that dead bodies are prone to suffering, and that mindless bodies will also suffer. The main drawback of such an objective approach is that judgements on suffering are made without considering the sufferer's viewpoint. In other words, the sufferer's rational judgement of his or her own suffering can be easily rejected or overruled. Mindless bodies would prove a difficult proposition in determining how they are suffering. The implication in clinical practice may be grave. If objectivity alone becomes permissible, then arguably treatments and interventions could be prescribed and delivered without consulting patients, even those who are *compos mentis*. In crude terms, this would be paternalism via the back door and a reminder of the much-criticised traditional medical model. Such practice would obviously fail to respect the wishes, needs, values and aspirations of the person, and would not be acceptable to nursing in general and in specialist areas (palliative care) in particular.

The second point, that suffering does not require mental consciousness, contradicts our earlier assertion that for suffering to occur it must take place at a mental level. Using the example of the girl discussed above, Van Hooft's position would support that this girl is suffering at the time of her abuse. The issue is not so much about whether the girl suffers or not, but at what point(s) in her life the suffering is experienced. There is a strong argument that suffering would be experienced at the time the girl becomes aware of her experiences, and only if these experiences affect her intactness as a person. Let us suppose there are two young girls growing up in these conditions of abuse and educational depravation. One of them realises that she is experiencing an abnormal and abusive upbringing, whilst the other, unaware of any abnormality, continues to consider her upbringing normal. It is more plausible to suggest that the girl who becomes aware of the abuse may suffer mentally from the experience, even when the bruises from the beatings are long healed. Arguably, the other would not experience any suffering.

Van Hooft also claims that being sick (the sick role) is a frustration on our being and constitutes a form of suffering. The frustration occurs at the deliberative (practical) level disrupting our life. This claim seems too stringent in that it ignores possible benefits within the sick role. Consider the case of a seventy-five year-old lonely man who lives in a noisy village and hardly affords to eat regular meals. His house is filthy, untidy, with no heating. He is admitted to hospital for assessment because he is not feeling well. In other words, his vegetative dimension is being frustrated, and according to Van Hooft, he would be suffering. It is absurd to suggest that this man, when admitted to hospital, is still suffering given his overall condition. There is a real possibility for contentedness and enjoyment for this lonely man who now finds himself in company, with regular meals and care. From recent correspondence with Van Hooft, he accepts the above critique, but maintains that suffering would still occur at the vegetative level. He writes, 'This is an interesting thought which I had not considered. There would be suffering at the vegetative level, of course, but contentedness at the higher levels. An interesting idea which confirms how complex we are'.

While this comment is welcome, it may suggest that in this situation, suffering may need to be 'weighted' against other benefits or feelings such as contentedness to arrive at the true nature or degree of the suffering, that is, 'net suffering'. In the case of the this lonely old man, arguably, the vegetative frustration would become insignificant in the face of what he has 'gained' by being admitted to hospital. The acknowledgement by Van Hooft that there is a higher level within a person, but without calling it the mental level, is an interesting one.

On being a person and the concept of suffering

Throughout this article, the term 'person' has been used without defining its meaning. Cassell (1992) acknowledges the difficulty of a precise definition, but claims that most people know what they mean when they say 'I am a person'. At a philosophical level, however, further discussion is needed to relate 'person' to 'suffering'. It is also important to explore how nursing defines a person and this will be attempted briefly. It is beyond the scope of this chapter to discuss what nursing is, and whether it is a science, an art or a practice.

Many philosophers, including Descartes (1591-1650), view the person in dualistic form of body and mind. Descartes argued that the mind and body were separate entities, hence the coining of the term 'Cartesian dualism' (Campbell, 1970; Collinson, 1987). However, Descartes's inability to prove the causal affect or interaction of these two entities gave ammunition to his critics. The body was viewed as material substance occupying space and not capable of thinking, while the mind was viewed as thinking, non-corporeal (intangible) and non-spatial. Substance can be defined as that which can exist independently, raising the question of whether the mind can exist independently too. Proponents of dualism would agree that it does, but stress the non-reducibility of the mind to body state. Edwards (2001) gives the example that the mind inhabits the body until death. This view of the person acknowledges suffering to occur at a mental level, therefore requiring mental consciousness. In other words, the mind is the essence and reality of persons.

The other view of person is offered as materialistic in which the person is viewed as matter. Materialism (Campbell, 1970) would incorporate everything that exists as matter, human beings included, thereby rejecting Cartesian dualism. According to Collinson, Spinoza (1632-1677) was one of the proponents of this view. On the other hand, proponents of monism upheld the doctrine that reality only consists of one substance, which can be matter or spiritual or even indefinite. Finally, some philosophers believe in idealism, which is the doctrine that reality ultimately consists of minds and ideas and that matter has no existence independently of our idea of it.

From these diverse perspectives, it also follows that suffering will be seen and subscribed to in diverse ways. What it is that suffers is one of the fundamental questions that needs to be addressed, as is the question of how the sufferer (person) is viewed. For example, if a person is viewed as materialistic, we can conclude that even mindless bodies suffer. Conversely, if a person is viewed in dualistic terms, it is logical to conclude that mindless bodies are not capable of experiencing suffering. Where a person is viewed in dualistic terms, in the case of Cartesian dualism, it also follows that the mind is the more fundamental of the two parts.

Nursing's view of person and suffering

The view of a person from a nursing perspective can be ascertained from nurse theorists. For purposes of this chapter, a brief overview of the work of Watson and Henderson, two prominent nurse theorists, will be given. According to Marriner-Tomey (1994), Henderson views the person as a biological human being, where the body and mind are inseparable. This view would therefore be sympathetic to the vegetative dimension. From this perspective, suffering can be said to occur without the mental consciousness, and accurately determined from the third-person (objective) perspective.

The second theorist to consider is Jean Watson who views a person as having a body and mind that are separable. Watson could be said to subscribe to the doctrine of dualism, after Descartes. However, the main difference is that Watson views the mind as existing without confinement to the physical sphere. The body would be viewed as being confined to space and time. From this, suffering could be argued to exist and be experienced subjectively. This then advances the view that suffering is best understood from the first-person perspective. There are other views in nursing considering the range of theories and theorists globally. These views tend to influence the way patients are cared for. It is clear that there is no consensus on how to view a person and this may also suggest a lack of consensus on the nature of suffering and its manifestations. It can be argued that with such a lack of consensus, the suffering that professionals purport to relieve may be different from what the patients actually experience.

Magnitude as a concept of suffering

The above concept is still in its infancy, and more work is needed to refine it before it catches on. However, it will suffice to give a brief overview here of how the concept would work. Comments and further discussion from interested readers would be welcome.

First, it is important to state that, through magnitude, the concept of suffering is best captured as a mental phenomenon and therefore involves mental consciousness. It also follows that suffering is a result of an experience one encounters, and therefore must be felt (Edwards, 2001), not only in the physical sense. If such suffering is to be true then the sufferer must feel it and be aware of it. This is the subjective concept of suffering, which is in line with most subjective models of care applied in palliative nursing.

This concept of suffering requires that two conditions, intensity (I) and duration (D), be present simultaneously. The collective term for ID is what is being referred to as magnitude (M); thus $I + D = M$. Intensity is based on pain (used broadly to encompass other negative experiences) being experienced and duration is the time that the pain is experienced. It is worth mentioning here that, exponentially, intensity comprises a fundamental or greater part of magnitude. It can be argued that I and D are two necessary conditions for suffering to occur.

However, the two entities should not be misconstrued as being necessary and sufficient conditions of suffering. Necessary and sufficient conditions are definitive and make something what it is and nothing else. In this concept, suffering is perceived and interpreted as different by various people due to its subjective nature. Using this approach, it may then be possible to describe the type of suffering depending on the two conditions. For example, where there is high intensity for a short period, the suffering could be described as acute. Where there is low intensity over a long period, the suffering could be described as chronic. In the case where both intensity and duration are medium, it is possible to describe the suffering as moderate. Obviously, there are 'grey areas', the in-betweens that cannot be clearly described, and here the reader is asked to use this idea as a guide until further work is concluded.

The brief explanation above gives a different position of capturing the essence of suffering from that offered by either Cassell or Van Hooft. This subjective concept of suffering can be used in nursing to provide meaningful relief from suffering. The fact that this view offers a subjective dimension would be more acceptable in palliative nursing (terminal illness) and therefore worthwhile defending here. The concept rejects suffering in mindless bodies but acknowledges that 'something else' happens, which can be inferred from the third-person perspective. As acknowledged earlier, magnitude as a concept of suffering will need revision, but in the meantime it hopefully offers a platform for discussion among healthcare professionals. It is hoped that with such discussion, more ideas will be generated and the concept refined.

Summary

The arguments and discussions offered so far confirm that the essence of suffering remains elusive. This elusiveness is due mainly to the different values, perspectives and meaning ascribed to suffering. However, there is also total agreement that suffering exists. It seems overwhelming that suffering is seen as a negative interpretation of the experience, often ignoring any positive outcomes such as personal growth, strengthened conviction, revised values, ambition, and an acquired ability to put things into their rightful perspectives.

Using the different perspectives of suffering presented by different researchers, three main themes emerge: objective, subjective and composite.

The objective attribute relies on the third person's inferences of someone else's suffering. Such an attribute relies heavily on the accuracy of the inferences and may not include the meaning, nor require mental consciousness. It is possible to measure this type of suffering quantitatively.

The subjective attribute relies on the first person's account, and is therefore unique and intuitive to that individual. This attribute accepts that suffering differs from person to person and therefore pays closer attention to the meaning attached to each suffering experience. Arguably, changing the meaning may relieve or exacerbate the suffering. It is important to emphasise that meaning is influenced by (among other things) a persons' culture, beliefs and values, past experiences, and unfulfilled aspirations. It is difficult to measure this type of suffering, and therefore professionals have to trust and believe in what the patient/sufferer tells them.

The composite attribute is a complex multidimensional perspective of suffering that also includes the two perspectives above. It acknowledges the psychological, emotional, physical, spiritual and interactional distress of a person in suffering. The assumption is that each of these dimensions can suffer separately but pervade the others (after Van Hooft, 1998). It therefore affects the 'intactness' of a person.

The implications of these attributes on interventions employed to relieve suffering are varied. The objective dimension would be permissible in mindless bodies, and would be a form of unacceptable paternalism in persons (ie. with a mind). On the other hand, the subjective dimension would rely on the professionals believing what the patient says about his or her suffering, and therefore simultaneously challenging the professionals' judgements, only if different from the patient's. The composite dimensions require meticulous assessment of the multiple aspects of a person, and then a decision on the most appropriate intervention to relieve the resultant suffering.

Conclusion

The question that probably remains unanswered in this chapter is how suffering can best be viewed in a palliative-care context. The three possible approaches above represent suffering from different perspectives, and also show the diversity of this complex phenomenon. The reader must appreciate that this phenomenon is not black and white, and these concluding thoughts are based on what I believe to be plausible from the discussion so far.

In palliative care, or in any other setting where professionals work in partnership with the patient, it is plausible to view suffering as a function of mental consciousness and that which is felt or experienced at the conscious level of persons. Here, the view of persons (that is, materialism or dualism) will have a huge bearing on how suffering is viewed and interpreted. For example, those who subscribe to the Cartesian dualism debate would strongly rely on the subjective view of suffering, where the patient determines his or her suffering. This approach seems more in line with the principles of palliative care, as opposed to the paternalistic view of caring.

If we accept the subjective view of suffering — which, according to the arguments so far, seems plausible in palliative care — we also have to reject suffering in unconscious patients and mindless bodies. Indeed, something happens in the unconscious patient, but we could not articulate 'it' as suffering, and perhaps another label is needed. In this case, the intervention could then be determined objectively (from a third-person perspective). When this perspective is used, it would be inaccurate to claim that the intervention is relieving suffering.

In the final analysis, it is important to understand theories, ethical and philosophical arguments, and defend them well professionally. Such indulgence will help us explore some of the more difficult existential questions encountered in our day-to-day work with dying patients. However, we must not lose sight of the patient's needs, wants and aspirations. More important is the experience the patients will have once we have cared for them. Carl Jung's (1875–1961) advice in relation to loss and bereavement can also be taken into palliative care:

> *Learn your theories as well as you can, but put them aside when touching the miracle of the living soul. Not theories, but your own creative individuality must decide.*

References

Campbell K (1970) *Body and Mind*. London: Macmillan

Cassell EJ (1991) *The Nature of Suffering: the Goals of Medicine*. Oxford: OUP

Cassell EJ (1992) The nature of suffering: physical, psychological, social and spiritual aspects. In: Starck P, McGovern J (eds) *The Hidden Dimension of Illness: Human Suffering*. New York: National League for Nursing Press

Collinson D (1987) *Fifty Major Philosophers: a Reference Guide*. London: Routledge

Edwards SD (1998) (ed) *Philosophical Issues in Nursing*. London: Macmillan

Edwards SD (2001) *Philosophy of Nursing: an Introduction*. Basingstoke: Palgrave

Edwards SD (2001) Three Concepts of Suffering. Unpublished paper

Forbes K, Faull C (1998) The principles of pain management. In: Faull C, Carter Y, Woof R (eds) *Handbook of Palliative Care*. Oxford: Blackwell Science

Frankl V (1962) *Man's Search for Meaning*. London: Hodder and Stoughton

Marriner-Tomey A (1994) *Nursing Theories and their Work*. Boston: Mosby

McKenna H (1997) *Nursing Theories and Models*. London: Routledge

Nyatanga B (2001) *Why Is It So Difficult to Die?* London: Quay Books

Rodgers BL, Cowles KV (1997) A conceptual foundation for human suffering in nursing and research. *J Adv Nurs* **25**: 1048–53

Van Hooft S (1998) Suffering and the goals of medicine. *Med Health Care Philos* **1**: 125–31

6

Social erosion or isolation in palliative care

Maxine Astley-Pepper

Hold my hand, oh hold it fast.
I am changing! — until at last
My hand in yours no more will change,
Though yours change on. You here, I there,
So hand in hand, twin-leafed despair —
I did not know death was so strange.

from 'The Child Dying' by Edwin Muir (Wollman, 1968)

Introduction

A personal experience, whilst working as a Macmillan Clinical Nurse Specialist, gave me the drive and impetus for this book and in particular this chapter.

This section will aim to explore the notion of social isolation and loneliness for those diagnosed with a life-threatening illness. The vignette described refers specifically to someone with acquired immunodeficiency syndrome (AIDS). However, the relevance to patients with cancer or other potentially terminal conditions is equally strong.

Loneliness is often well-hidden from others, in accordance with the old adage that one may be with family, friends or colleagues, yet still have a profound sense of loneliness or 'aloneness.' The health professional is in a unique position to identify and address this situation. It will, however, require effective communication skills and self-awareness. The sense of loneliness and isolation may be insidious and the risk of depression increased. This process may become a vicious cycle if left untreated.

Vignette

I was caring for a twenty-seven year-old man with AIDS, whom I will refer to as Mark. He was married with two children, and had endured the perils of haemophilia all his life.

A contaminated blood transfusion caused, for him, the most traumatic emotional fragmentation possible. His frightened wife left, taking the children with her, he lost his job, and friends seemed to just disappear. He moved to live with his parents. His mother, a nurse, dealt with all his daily physical care and together she and his father tried to manage his emotional distress.

Excuses as to why people no longer visited the house soon became problematic and Mark slowly withdrew from conversation and interaction with those who did call. He once told me that he felt like a leper. This phrase was also used by a patient in a study by Taylor (2001), showing how patients report feeling 'on their own' following a diagnosis of cancer. Feelings of exclusion, anticipated changes in themselves (physical and emotional), and feeling 'dirty' were widely reported within this research. Mark's drastically altered appearance distressed him so much that he refused to have mirrors in the room, and the curtains were closed so that he could not see his reflection in the glass. Price (2000) associates this loss of self-esteem to the patient's perceived loss of control, and suggests that society equates such dysfunction with deterioration in other faculties, such as mental ability.

The aim of this chapter is to explore the notion of social isolation and erosion often reported by those who have received a diagnosis of cancer. This may be a perceived or real phenomenon that manifests itself from the very instant the individual is diagnosed (Taylor, 2001).

Historically, cancer — and even just the word itself — evokes fear, uncertainty and fatalism in most people, not necessarily just in those who have the disease. Immediately, there is a sense of reduced life expectancy (see *Chapter 7*); for many, the word 'cancer' is almost like a death knell.

Mellor (1993) suggests that in today's modern, health-conscious society, death itself is 'hidden' and therefore a diagnosis that exposes our vulnerability and morbidity may have profound implications for our social structures. Given this, one can begin to understand why, in our quest for eternal youth and longevity, individuals may shy away from interacting with those who are dying, as this may interfere with their perception of everlasting life.

In trying to understand the process of social disengagement, behavioural psychologists have explored the ageing process on which to base this phenomenon (see Gross, 2001). Cumming and Henry (1961) did a longitudinal study looking at the process by which the individual mutually withdraws from society, influenced by retirement, children leaving home, death of a spouse and friends, etc. As a consequence, their roles in life are reduced and the need to comply with rules and regulations lessened; in effect, there is a loss of control. Furthermore, the healthy older person adapts and embraces this phase of their life, in preparation for their eventual death (Cumming, 1975). In contrast to the idea that the older person disengages from society, Havighurst (1964) and Maddox (1964) have claimed that society withdraws from the older person.

However, later studies dispute this concept and Bee (1994) suggests that relationships and roles are essential components for emotional balance in the ageing person. As cancer and life-limiting illness may affect people of any age, how then may we better understand the process of disengagement that occurs for them?

The impact of the diagnosis may affect the individual in many ways and losses may include:

- employment — early retirement, loss of job
- financial — loss, reduced income
- roles at home, parent, carer, provider
- roles in society — eg. status, clubs, activities
- dignity — due to surgery, treatment or disease process
- relationships — professional, personal, sexual (see *Chapter 9*)
- confidence, self-esteem
- control — perceived or real
- future
- hope.

These losses mirror those associated with the effects of ageing, so the theories appear to be equally applicable to the palliative-care patient. Indeed, they may also bear relevance to the grieving process, whereby disengagement, aimlessness, apathy and despair are stages that the bereaved are liable to experience (Parkes, 1996).

Society's attitude toward disease has a significant impact on the 'journey' for the individual. In the past, people with cancer were often kept isolated from society as many falsely believed — and still do — that cancer is contagious. This belief only serves to ostracise the individual further, and may be interpreted as 'social death'. An example of this is the person with AIDS, often shunned by their contemporaries and family members who avoid physical contact and obsessively clean eating and drinking utensils in an attempt to avoid 'contamination' (Open University, 1998). Whilst health education and information strives to dispel such myths, and patients may no longer believe that they are contagious, their deterioration and reduced social interaction leads them to feeling that 'it is as if they are contagious' (Price, 2000). This in turn may develop into a profound state of loneliness, shame and self-hatred (Brown and McKenna, 1999).

Social isolation and loneliness

Loneliness is the feeling of being alone in spite of longing to be with others. The lonely person experiences a sense of utter aloneness, often accompanied by aimlessness and boredom.

Brown and McKenna (1999)

For the patient with a life-threatening illness, loneliness may be a profound reality. As for the patient with a communicable disease, society has its own way of creating social isolation for an individual with cancer, often as a result of anxiety, fear and ignorance. For Mark, the name of his illness alone, AIDS, evoked panic amidst his own family and indeed for some of his professional carers. In fact, some professionals refused to attend him. This also included funeral directors who were contacted by Mark when he was trying to make his funeral plans. He was so despondent following these rejections that he visibly withdrew from communicating with others and became uninterested in his surroundings, eventually becoming completely anhedonic.

This case was all the more poignant for Mark and his family because he had had no control over the disease that required frequent transfusions (haemophilia) or the contamination by the infected blood (AIDS). He had been given a life-limiting illness by the profession that was there to care for and protect him. This may have also compounded his reluctance to communicate with doctors and nurses and accelerated the process of disengagement. Within the gay community, there appears to be a network for mutual support and understanding for those with AIDS that does not obviously exist within the heterosexual community. Maybe this lack of understanding and exposure to those with AIDS compounds the myths and fears surrounding this relatively new disease.

In writing about AIDS patients specifically, Kirkpatrick (1993) suggests that fear itself is a communicable disease, and that professionals and politicians have an obligation to ensure that every individual is given equal consideration and respect. Kirkpatrick (1993) quotes Clarke (1988):

… structural changes in society had been of such an order that society's own immune defences are suppressed… while the AIDS virus is an opportunistic infection of the human body, 'AIDS the syndrome' can be regarded as an opportunistic infection of the lowered immune system of the social structure itself.

This statement suggests that there is a lack of cohesion, or a sense of disempowerment, within society to enable those with life-limiting illness to be adequately supported or indeed acknowledged as belonging to the wider community. Supporting this notion, Dicks (1999) has reported a lack of palliative-care support for non-cancer patients.

Patients with cancer may experience feelings of aloneness within their own family network. In order to support them, health professionals, particularly the palliative-care team, have the opportunity to focus on this aspect of care delivery.

In this new millennium of advanced technology, therapeutic interventions and virtual eradication of some diseases, death is no longer deemed to be an inevitable life phase, but appears to have been sanitised and often viewed as a medical failure. This may partly explain why doctors sometimes struggle to admit to patients that they have no further treatment options with which to treat their disease.

Health professionals are uneasy about giving life-altering news and so, in the case of cancer, for example, such news has for decades been couched in 'easier to bear' euphemisms, such as 'lump' or 'growth', or in technical terms, such as 'malignancy', 'tumour' or 'neoplasm' (Open University, 1998). A sense of personal failure may overwhelm the physician, rendering him/her incapable of preventing the patient from experiencing the profound sense of alienation, isolation and loneliness that the 'dying phase' can bring with it.

The sense of failure, fear and shame

The communication networks and media coverage, reaching a worldwide audience, brings the reality of cancer into our everyday domain. Unfortunately, the interpretation of the dying process is often depicted as a battle. Newspaper obituary features often include statements such as:

> *A brave and courageous lady who battled to the end.*
>
> *Leicester Mercury* (2004)

> *My darling… you fought for life with courage until the very end.*
>
> *Leicester Mercury* (2004)

> *After much suffering bravely borne, over many years.*
>
> *Evening Telegraph* (2004)

The negative, defeated connotations of these statements — however well-meaning — only compound a sense that dying is indeed the ultimate 'failure', for both patients and professionals alike. Personal memorial tributes often mirror these sentiments and could lead to relatives feeling that their loved one has indeed failed them and maybe didn't try hard enough to overcome their disease. These feelings may distort memories and impede the grieving process, as opposed to those for whom death is seen as a natural progression of the life 'timeline'.

Similarly, the suggestion of being courageous may serve to 'disable' patients when they wish to speak of their fear. Dixon *et al* (1996) state that fear is most profound at the time of disease recurrence. Weisman and Worden (1986), however, suggest that there is no real difference between this patient group and those at initial diagnosis. This situation may prohibit the patient from disclosing how they feel and lead to the internalisation of their fears and anxieties. This may be borne from the patients' strong desire to protect their family or indeed themselves.

A recent quality of life research study supports this protective gesture in palliative-care patients who felt they were 'protecting their loved one from pain by not openly acknowledging how ill they were'. Furthermore, these patients would 'go along with the carer's goals even when they actually believed them to be unrealistic' (McLoughlin, 2002).

Consider, then, the internal stress of keeping up this façade and the effect that this may have on the individual. The patient may be experiencing a type of 'collusion with self', oscillating between acceptance of the poor prognosis and denial of it (Field and Copp, 1999). The impact of this emotional subterfuge on the individual may result in clinical depression.

Depression

Social isolation for the cancer patient may be compounded by the onset of depression, of which there is a high incidence among the terminally ill. Sadly, this can often go undiagnosed (McVey, 1998; Payne, 1998).

Given that the literature suggests that social isolation is part of the transitional process, and that cancer patients may become withdrawn, prompt assessment and treatment of depression is required. Therefore, professionals need to see 'beyond the disease' and explore the patient's anxieties and fears in order to prevent spiralling dissociation. Palliative-care nurses are proficient at recognising psychological distress in patients, and detecting and reporting signs of guilt, hopelessness and worthlessness (McVey, 1998).

McVey (1998) states: 'An important aspect of the treatment of the depressed patient is social interaction'. This supports the earlier suggestion that professionals are in a unique position to encourage patients and help maintain their position and integration in society. The world of the patient will be permanently changed by their illness, their concept of time, future and hope altered forever. The professional team has the skills to try to understand this new world without actually entering it with the patient (see *Chapter 3*).

This chapter has highlighted the way in which some patients may suppress their own feelings and adopt a pretence of well-being in order to protect others. However, they may still be prone to depression, which has three main manifestations:

- somatic — loss of energy, anorexia, altered weight, sleep disturbances
- cognitive — feelings of worthlessness, failure, guilt, apathy
- affective — sadness and crying.

Moreover, any of these symptoms may be experienced by the dying patient, distinguishing clinical depression from the normal symptoms of the disease process (eg. anorexia, sadness, fatigue). Identifying true clinical depression is not easy and detection and diagnosis of depression remains poor (Payne, 1998). Furthermore, Payne suggests that people who show persistent, severe changes in mood that prevent them from participating in day-to-day life are clinically depressed, and that this can be compounded by anxiety. Potentially, a vicious cycle could occur, whereby patients are unable to communicate their innermost thoughts and fears. Patients need to discuss their feelings, a point made by McVey (1998):

Allowing the patient to express their feelings, fears and anger and listening in a non-judgemental manner helps to reduce the patient's fears of being perceived as weak.

Health professionals have a unique and challenging opportunity to care for the cancer patient, or indeed any individual with a life-limiting disease. They have not only a duty of care, but also a duty to share their expertise, knowledge and self.

Health professionals' responsibility

Palliative-care nurses provide excellent physical care and sensitive support to dying patients (Price, 2000). However, there is much still to be done to support the patient, for whom altered body image and subsequent loss of self-esteem and control is profound. For example, Mark underwent devastating altered body image due to the ravages of AIDS, including dramatic weight loss, hair loss, loss of bodily functions, and the development of Karposi's sarcoma. This previously 'acceptable' man had become abhorrent to others. His self-esteem plummeted and his self-image was further damaged when some of his carers displayed fear of the disease by not wanting to touch him with ungloved hands, and did not stay with him long enough to assess his emotional turmoil.

He experienced society's disengagement, probably due to fear, anxiety and maybe ignorance of the disease itself. Preparation for this type of reaction is difficult, for both patient and professionals alike, and, for many, it may elicit a response to otherwise suppressed opinions, preconceptions or prejudices.

Preparing patients (at the point of diagnosis) for the reactions they may experience along their disease trajectory is crucial if their quality of life is to be optimised. Moreover, given Mellor's (1993) theory of loneliness and society's attitude toward the dying, health professionals, and indeed the patient, are part of that society and may struggle with their own interpretation and concept of death. Elias (1985) suggests that a meaningful death is dependant upon the individual's memory, experience and image of death within their own culture. Also, the dying process will be greatly influenced by the person's ability to set and achieve goals along the way. This may be difficult if the person's professional carers are struggling with their own feelings and social attitudes.

Brown and McKenna (1999) recommend that nurses wishing to provide a truly holistic approach to patient care should pay more attention to 'how they see a patient', and that they should:

reconsider their approach to caring for the psychosocial needs of patients, focus more on assessing each individualised experience and aim to plan care to reduce the negative impact of loneliness.

If practitioners, then, do not communicate honestly and openly with patients about their diseases and prognoses, they are denying reality in order to protect themselves, rather than their patients, from the truth. This adaptive behaviour mirrors the constructivist approach to reality, whereby a person defines truth as it exists in their individual mind and not as it is known as proven fact (Rolfe *et al*, 2001). This in turn may influence the patient and family, and lead to a totally distorted view of the illness. Indeed, many professionals will be able to recall discussions with patients who have received a terminal disease diagnosis, and whose recollection of the conversation with the doctor bears little resemblance to what was really said. This may be the patient's way of defining the truth in order to maintain an ability to cope, or indeed, to prevent the loneliness and anxiety that may be triggered by an uncertain future (Price, 1999).

For some, repeated truth-telling will not alter this mechanism, as the patient's interpretation will always be, for them, the reality. This denial of reality may prove frustrating for the care-givers, but they should avoid being 'drawn in' to this deception and maintain their own self-awareness. If not, as the true reality of the situation unfurls, there may be an irreparable breakdown in the therapeutic relationship between professional and patient. Furthermore, the important role of the professional as advocate and facilitator may be stifled.

Professionals must be mindful that as a consequence of the behaviour of one professional, the patient may have a mistrust of the profession as a whole at a time when their needs and vulnerability are increasing. They may be thrust into further isolation, not knowing what the truth really is, or whom they can trust. To possess self-awareness and effective communication skills is essential if the practitioner is to be truly congruent with the patient.

Self-awareness

The need to become more self-aware, particularly through reflective practice, is a recurring theme in current nursing literature, as is looking at behaviour as well as practice to support professional competence (Boud *et al*, 1985). Indeed, nursing and medical education holds reflection as an integral part of the learning process. The governing body for nurses, The Nursing and Midwifery Council (2002a), requires every nurse and midwife to reflect on practice in order to develop towards becoming an expert practitioner. This process of examining practice may challenge nurses' own assumptions and beliefs, develop enhanced listening skills and change practice accordingly, moving towards a more truly holistic approach to patient care (Burnard, 1995; Durgahee, 1996).

Spall and Johnson (1997) observed that nurses' own fears surrounding caring for the dying were significantly reduced when this process was undertaken. However, the need for emotional support for palliative-care nurses was clearly identified. This upholds the notion that caring for the dying patient has an emotional impact on the professionals involved. Atkins (2000) suggests that reflection enables practitioners to develop and evaluate their thinking and practice. Maybe during this process for developing self-awareness, the individual may be empowered to redefine existing thoughts and behaviours that have hitherto inhibited practice, to deliver effective, quality patient care. This can only improve professional and personal development and enhance communication skills.

Communication

> *It appeared that the main reason causing their isolation was the general inhibition to communicate about cancer.*
>
> Taylor (2001)

The way we communicate our feelings to the dying patient is crucial — our body language, in particular, 'speaks' volumes. A patient once reported that after his consultant had told him that there was nothing more that could be done to treat his disease, the consultant no longer included the patient in his ward round. He passed by the bed without a glance. He was indeed 'telling him' that he was no longer there, that he was unimportant and invisible ('like I was already gone'). The patient became withdrawn and refused to communicate with the nursing staff and his condition rapidly deteriorated. This patient was vulnerable and felt that he had been 'left to die' by the professionals caring for him. The reaction of the doctor (in this scenario) could be a catalyst for both physical and psychosocial deterioration in the patient (Taylor, 1993).

Furthermore, this behaviour contradicts the notion of total care delivery and indeed fails to address the basic physical and psychosocial needs of each human being — ie. to belong, to be loved, and to search for a sense of meaning (Maslow, 1987). These needs are as relevant and important to the dying as they are to the living.

The role of the professional is to facilitate this process and support the patient through this difficult period of adjustment with honesty, openness, tenderness and caring — and, above all, to show that they are 'present' with the individual (see *Chapter 4*). In doing so, they are communicating that the person means something and that they are still important. Although the journey into death is a lonely one, and one that cannot be shared, reassurance that one is not alone during this process is essential.

Holistic care delivery, then, should enable the professionals to address the impact not only of the disease, but also of their own words and deeds on their patients. Studies suggest that the news of disease recurrence, subsequent deterioration, and threat of death may evoke intense fear within the individual. For the patient, this fear may equate to a lack of courage that had been expected of them by their relatives, and ultimately lead to a sense of failure (Dixon *et al*, 1996).

Professionals need to be aware of the impact that this situation may have on the individual and the family — eg. depression, breakdown in communication, and despair. There is a real opportunity here for the professional carers to support the patient and the family. Skilled communication and encouragement are essential in helping preserve fragile relationships at this vulnerable time — for example, including the patient's views in his care for as long as possible and facilitating open dialogue between patient and relatives in a supportive manner (Nebauer *et al*, 1996).

Bertero (1998) suggests that the patient's interaction with nursing and medical staff is crucial in facilitating the understanding of, and the adjustment to, the new situation that the transition from the treatable to the palliative phase requires. The patient will also undergo a complete re-definition of his or her place in society, and may temporarily lose sight of familiar frames of reference within it. The individual will require accurate and honest information in order to modify behaviour and 'make sense' of the new situation.

As the future for each cancer patient is unclear, they may experience several transitional phases during their disease trajectory. Challenges to their personal constructs and values may affect communication and compliance. They will have a heightened awareness and sensitivity to the behaviour of others, paying particular attention to the non-verbal language and interactions between health professionals. Therefore, all the members of the palliative-care multidisciplinary team need to be aware of their own behaviour and attitude, and how these may affect the patient and outcome. Above all, showing an understanding of the patient's sense of aloneness and isolation is essential if they are to receive skilled and appropriate support (Bertero, 1998; Taylor, 2001).

In addition to body language, patients will initially see the reaction to their physical appearance mirrored in the face of the beholder, so it is essential that health professionals have awareness of this response. Treatment-induced hair loss, cachexia, skin lesions and fungating wounds are just a few of the many changes that can affect an individual. Relationships with others may be profoundly affected, particularly between partners (see *Chapter 9*), compounding the existing loneliness and isolation that the patient may be feeling. The first face-to-face encounter between a patient and a health professional is the one that both will remember. How they were received and accepted by the health professional is vital to the patient. At this early stage, eye contact and expression can be the catalyst for success or failure of the therapeutic relationship.

Conclusion

In drawing on personal experience, anecdotes and relevant literature, this chapter has, I hope, highlighted the issue of social isolation in the context of cancer and palliative care. This is a hidden aspect that we as individuals are not always able to 'see' or acknowledge — ie. fear, loneliness or depression in others. Many patients are able to mask their innermost feelings and hide deep-seated emotions from those who care for them, so the responsibility of the health professional is to heighten their own awareness of these emotions and alert others to them. For some reading this chapter, the hidden aspects discussed may actually be obvious; however, for many, the focus may be the treatment modalities, physical comfort and day-to-day care of the patient. One can never point out the obvious too often.

Healthcare professionals are in a unique (and often unenviable) position in the care of patients with cancer or life-limiting illnesses. They have the opportunity to influence and empower the individual by offering support, understanding and timely, accurate information. Professional care-givers have an obligation to try to enter the world of the patient and facilitate and coordinate a therapeutic relationship with each individual. This is the most important phase in the life of any patient — and there are no 'second chances'. Through skilled communication, awareness and acceptance of our own personal attitudes, we may need to re-configure our behaviour to the individual in order to understand their perspective and behaviour, without compromising our own selfhood.

Caring for others, particularly in the terminal phase of their illness, is not without its own demands and, through heightened self-awareness, our own vulnerability may also be exposed. Therefore, support mechanisms, such as reflective practice, clinical supervision and peer support, are essential to prevent disengagement occurring within the care setting.

The ability for a disease to infiltrate every facet of an individual is astounding. Ironically, that same disease may equally affect those associated (in a caring role) with the patient in an insidious, sometimes hidden manner. In this scenario, the care-giver may also collude and deny, become depressed and feel worthless. The latter may be due to the inability to cure, or feeling inadequate to deal with the complex issues at hand.

Whilst, medically, there may be little more that can be done for the individual, the health professional should never underestimate the impact and power of attendance, or of 'presence of self'. A detailed account of presencing can be found in *Chapter 4*.

References

Atkins S (2000) Developing underlying skills in the move toward reflective practice. In: Burns S, Bulman C (eds) *Reflective Practice in Nursing: the Growth of the Professional Practitioner*. Oxford: Blackwell Science

Bee H (1994) Lifespan developement. In: Gross R (1996) (ed) *Psychology – the Science of Mind and Behaviour*. 3rd edition. London: Hodder & Stoughton

Bertero CM (1998) Transition to becoming a leukaemia patient: or putting up barriers which increase social isolation. *Eur J Cancer Care (Engl)* **7**: 40–6

Boud D, Keogh R, Walker D (1985) *Reflection: Turning Experience into Learning*. London: Kagan

Brown R, McKenna HP (1999) Concept analysis of loneliness in dying patients. *Int J Palliat Nurs* **5**(2): 90–7

Burnard P (1995) *Learning Human Skills*. Oxford: Butterworth Heinemann

Clarke P (1988) AIDS: medicine, politics and society. In: Kirkpatrick B (1993) (ed) *AIDS: Sharing the Pain – Guide for Carers*. 2nd edition. London: Dartman, Longman & Todd

Cumming E, Henry WE (1961) Growing old: the process of disengagement. In: Gross R (1996) (ed) *Psychology – the Science of Mind and Behaviour*. 3rd edition. London: Hodder & Stoughton

Cumming E (1975) Engagement with an old theory. In: Gross R (1996) (ed) *Psychology – the Science of Mind and Behaviour*. 3rd edition. London: Hodder & Stoughton

Dixon R, Lee-Jones C, Humphries G (1996) Psychological reactions to cancer recurrence. *Int J Palliat Nurs* **2**(1): 19–21

Durgahee T (1996) Reflective practice: linking theory and practice in palliative care nursing. *Int J Palliat Nurs* **2**(1): 22–5

Elias N (1985) *The Loneliness of the Dying*. Oxford: Basil Blackford

Evening Telegraph (2004) **11 Feb**: 16

Field D, Copp G (1999) Communication and awareness about dying in the 1990s. In: McLoughlin PA (2002) (ed) Community specialist palliative care: experiences of patients and carers. *Int J Palliat Nurs* **8**(7): 344–53

Gross RD (2001) (ed) *Psychology — the Science of Mind and Behaviour.* 4th edition. London: Edward Arnold

Havighurst RJ (1964) Stages of vocational development. In: Gross R (1996) (ed) *Psychology – the Science of Mind and Behaviour.* 3rd edition. London: Hodder & Stoughton

Kirkpatrick B (1993) *AIDS: Sharing the Pain – Guide for Carers.* 2nd edition. London: Dartman, Longman & Todd

Leicester Mercury (2004) **Feb 11**: 38–9

Maddox GL (1964) Disengagement theory: a critical evaluation. In: Gross R (1996) (ed) *Psychology – the Science of Mind and Behaviour.* 3rd edition. London: Hodder & Stoughton

Maslow AH (1987) Motivation and personality. In: Spall B, Callis S (1997) (eds) *Loss, Bereavement and Grief: a Guide to Effective Caring.* Cheltenham: Stanley Thornes

McLoughlin PA (2002) Community specialist palliative care: experiences of patients and carers. *Int J Palliat Nurs* **8**(7): 344–53

McVey P (1998) Depression among the palliative care oncology population. *Int J Palliat Nurs* **4**(2): 86–93

Mellor P (1993) Death in high modernity: the contemporary presence and absence of death. In: Brown R, McKenna HP (1999) Conceptual analysis of loneliness in dying patients. *Int J Palliat Nurs* **5**(2): 90–7

Nebauer M, Prior D, Berggen L, Haberecht J, Ku M, Mitchell A, Davies E (1996) Nurses' perceptions of palliative care nursing. *Int J Palliat Nurs* **2**(1): 26–35

Nursing and Midwifery Council (NMC) (2002a) *Prep and You: Maintaining Your Registration: Standards for Education Following Registration.* London: NMC

Parkes CM (1996) *Bereavement Studies of Grief in Adult Life.* 3rd edition. London: Routledge

Payne S (1998) Depression in palliative care patients: a literature review. Int J Palliat Nurs **4**(4): 184–91

Price B (2000) Altered body image: managing social encounters. *Int J Palliat Nurs* **6**(4): 179–185

Spall R, Johnson M (1997) Experiential exercises in palliative care training. *Int J Palliat Nurs* **3**(4): 222–6

Taylor C (2001) Patients' experiences of 'feeling on their own' following a diagnosis of colo-rectal cancer: a phenomenological approach. *Int J Nurs Stud* 651–61

Taylor EJ (1993) Factors associated with meaning in life among people with recurrent cancer. *Oncol Nurs Forum* **20**(9): 1399–1405

Open University (1998) *Death and Dying Workbook 2: Preparation for Death.* Kent: Thanet Press

Weisman AD, Worden JW (1986) The emotional impact of recurrent cancer. *J Psychol Oncol* **3**(4): 5–16

Wollman M (1968) *Seven Themes in Modern Verse.* London: Harrap & Co

7

Hidden aspects of psychosocial care

Helen Walsh

Introduction

Psychosocial care seeks to address the psychological and emotional well-being of patients and their families (NCHSPCS, 1997). Focusing on issues such as self-esteem, communication, social functioning, relationships and insight into the illness, psychosocial care helps the individual and family's adaptation to living with the illness, and its associated consequences (Hughes, 1999). This involves working with the individual as a person in their own right, whilst recognising their role within the family, individual family members and with the family unit as a whole. Psychosocial care aims to enhance the well-being, confidence and social functioning of the family without using formal psychological methods such as counselling or psychotherapy (NCHSPCS, 1997). Such is the importance of psychological care that the NICE guidance (2004) recommendations include:

- Assessment of needs at key points in the patient pathway.
- The referral for specialist psychological care for those with significant levels of distress.
- The ability of all staff directly responsible for patient care to offer emotional support.
- The adequate training of and support for staff providing psychological care.

The purpose of this chapter is to explore the hidden aspects of psychosocial care. Before we can do this, we need to establish what we mean by the term 'hidden' in relation to psychosocial care. The term 'hidden' is perhaps, in this context, more difficult to explain since it's very meaning is to 'put or keep out of sight' (Thompson, 1995). This would suggest that the hidden aspects of psychosocial care are those topics or themes that one does not want to discuss or bring out into the open. The sorts of issues that immediately spring to mind are perhaps related to areas of sexuality, spirituality or relationship difficulties. These areas are indeed difficult to address and may well be considered to remain 'hidden' (Lugton, 2002; Sutherland and Gamlin, 1999; Johnson, 1998). This maybe more as a result of the inexperience or lack of skills on the part of the health and social care workers than a direct indication of the true hidden aspects of psychosocial care.

Whilst it would be convenient to attempt to isolate the psychosocial issues from other aspects of care, in reality, this is neither possible nor realistic. This is because psychosocial care is only one of the four components that make up the total care model for palliative care (*Figure 7.1*). Since psychosocial, practical, physical and spiritual aspects of care are all closely interwoven, the boundaries between them are ambiguous and cannot be clearly defined. Whilst the specific purpose of some physical interventions is to improve the patient's emotional and psychological state — for example, administering anti-depressants — all physical contact has emotional and psychological consequences (NCHSPCS, 1997). At a very basic level, even just washing, shaving, cleaning teeth and combing hair can make someone feel better about themselves (Jeffrey, 2003).

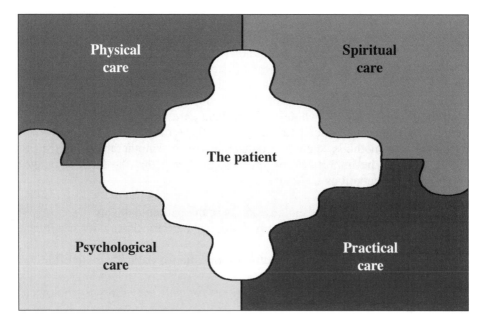

Figure 7.1: The patient in palliative care (adapted from NCHSPCS, 1997)

The fact that the psychosocial aspect of care is so difficult to extract begs the question as to whether such care really exists. If it does not, then considerable time and energy is being spent inappropriately seeking to address something which does not need addressing. This argument questions the fundamental principles of the palliative-care movement. Since its inception, it has been committed to re-establishing a holistic view of the patient and his/her care within the science of medicine, which seeks to control the physical effects of the disease itself (Hockley, 1997). In her very early work, Cicely Saunders emphasised the need for good physical care to be combined with psychological and spiritual assistance (Saunders, 1958). Without total care and its psychosocial element, palliative care is no longer a medical and nursing specialty. A useful way to illustrate the complexities and interconnectedness of the four components of total care is through the use of a case study.

George was a seventy-three year-old man with metastatic prostate cancer. He was married to Mary for over fifty years and they had two grown-up children who lived nearby. Whilst George was troubled with pain, constipation and mild nausea, these symptoms were reasonably well controlled with medication. Since the news that George's disease had escaped hormonal control, Mary had taken on the role of decision-maker, excluding him from even simple everyday choices. Mary said this was because she did not want him 'worrying' when time was so precious. He described it as 'being wrapped up in cotton wool'. As a result, George began to feel undermined, as though his purpose and contribution to the family were no longer important or valued (Hughes, 1999).

A very practical man, George was determined to 'put his house in order' and recognised the need for him to make a will. Although he wanted and was able to make the appointment with the solicitor, he needed considerable emotional and psychological support from his son to enable him to achieve this goal. While George would not describe himself as a religious man, he was surprised at the depth of his emotional response following a conversation with a neighbour about the purpose of life. He said afterwards that this conversation had made him think about how he viewed himself and the things he really valued.

Whilst this case study concentrates on the patient and family, the knock-on effect that care in one domain has on another is equally pertinent when professionals are involved. The benevolent, paternalistic attitude traditionally inherent in health care often results in professionals making decisions on the patient's behalf (Alexander, 2001; Sheldon, 1997). If they are capable of making or at least contributing to these decisions and are excluded, patients can, as in the case study above, begin to feel undermined as people.

Each family member will react and adapt differently to living with the diagnosis of a life-threatening illness (Hughes, 1999; McIntyre, 1999). These responses depend on the individual personalities of those concerned, the nature of the relationships (husband to wife, mother to son, etc.) and the quality of the existing relationships before the diagnosis (Hughes, 1999). People will also come to terms with the diagnosis in their own time (Buckman, 2001).

Since it is impractical and impossible to isolate its delivery from the other aspects of care (NCHSPCS, 1997), all healthcare professionals involved in caring for people with palliative care needs, irrespective of their discipline, are going to provide psychosocial care (Walker *et al*, 2003). Indeed, one cannot go and 'do' psychosocial care in the same way that one can go and 'do' a bed bath (physical care); undertake a home assessment (social care); or administer a religious rite (spiritual care). In its broadest sense, every contact with a patient and family offers the opportunity to care for their psychosocial needs (NCHSPCS, 1997). Effective psychological care, which is well thought-out, can be of benefit for all patients (Becker, 2001). The challenge is for us to recognise and maximise all opportunities in order to give good psychosocial care.

This chapter looks beyond the obvious and to discover what is happening below the surface for the patient and family at the psychosocial level.

The obvious aspects of psychosocial palliative care

Any individual (and their family), either newly diagnosed or those living with a life-threatening illness, are going to experience psychosocial difficulties, although the precise nature and severity of these needs will depend upon the individuals concerned (Hughes; 1999; NCHSPCS, 1997; Sheldon, 1997). The newly diagnosed patient and family suddenly find themselves robbed of the vague long-term future we all believe ourselves to have (Hughes, 1999; Lugton, 1999; Parkes, 1971). The exact nature of this future, or the 'assumptive world' as Parkes (1971) describes it, depends on the individual perceptions of previous experiences, expectations and plans. Future certainties which have been anticipated and planned for may still happen, but will do so in the absence of a key player. Fear, anxiety and dread replace the often unacknowledged feelings of anticipation and expectation of our future lives (Becker, 2001; Hughes, 1999; Sheldon, 1997).

Following the diagnosis, the family unit begins the uncertain and frightening journey of living with the disease (McIntyre, 1999; Lugton, 1999). The precise nature of that journey depends on the disease, its stage and its management, and indeed to a large extent on the family making it (Hughes, 1999). Surgery, radiotherapy and chemotherapy may be used in isolation or in combination. Each brings with it its own problems and threats to the individual undergoing the treatment and to those who love that person. For the patient, the illness and its treatments may cause pain, anorexia, hair loss, weight loss and dependence and usually involves the taking of multiple medications (Hughes, 1999). All treatments require time and as a consequence the patient and the family lose time from their normal lives in terms of absence from work, day-to-day activities and social interactions. As the individual is bombarded on a physical level in an attempt to cure or control the disease, on a psychological level, he or she is coming to terms with the loss of who they were and struggling to accept who they have become.

Having someone with a life-threatening illness within the family tends to affect all its members (Becker, 2001). Whilst other family members rarely experience the physical trauma of treatment, they too have to face their own psychosocial challenges (Sheldon, 2003). For example, partners may need to take on the roles their loved one can no longer fulfil, which in turn challenges their own concept of who they are (Hughes, 1999). Children see their role models changing as relationships between the adults alter in response to the effects of the disease and its management. Household routine can sometimes be dramatically affected as life now revolves around hospital visits and chemotherapy regimes, and the home becomes invaded by professional strangers ranging from district nurses to home helps. For many families, the financial effects of having an ill person can be catastrophic, resulting in considerable changes to the family's lifestyle (Sheldon, 2003; Becker, 2001; McIntyre, 1999).

These psychosocial issues are fairly obvious and any health or social care worker worth their salt would want to explore how the individual and family are coping with these issues surrounding the illness. Often, help can be given simply by offering space and privacy for them all to talk about their feelings, either individually or as a family (Jeffrey, 2003; Neuberger, 1999).

Hidden aspects of psychosocial care

But what exactly are we trying to do as we attempt to help people deal with the psychosocial issues caused by their illness? Is there anything that can help us understand what is happening? One framework which might be of help is the Hierarchy of Human Needs proposed by Albert Maslow (1970) (*Figure 7.2*). Maslow (1970) suggested that the motivation underpinning all human behaviour can be organised within a hierarchy, which he conceptualised as the triangle of human need. This triangle is divided into five sections, the bottom two of which address our social, physiological and environmental needs, while the top three sections are concerned with the more complex needs relating to psychological and emotional issues. According to Maslow (1970) until our basic needs (food, shelter, warmth) are met, we are unable to pursue our needs for security and safety. Likewise, until we feel safe, we cannot begin to identify with others, seek their acceptance, or search for suitable individuals with whom we would want to build supportive relationships.

As the needs within each level of the triangle are fulfilled or satisfied, so we are able to progress and begin to meet the challenges offered by the next stage. This process continues until we reach the pinnacle of the triangle, which is the point of such personal growth and development that we attain what Maslow (1970) describes as 'self actualisation'. When we arrive at this point, we have completely fulfilled our individual potential. There is some discussion, however, as to whether it is possible ever to reach this pinnacle because how can we know when we have reached our full potential and have no further scope to develop and grow? (Gross, 2001) The answer to this question is, however, outside the scope of this chapter.

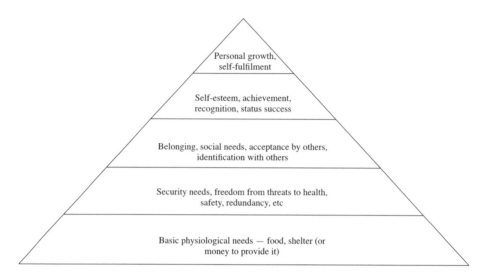

Figure 7.2: Maslow's 'triangle of human needs' (Marson *et al*, 1992)

Of more relevance is the exploration of how the triangle of human needs helps us understand the hidden aspects of psychosocial care in palliative care. As described above, Maslow (1970) argued that we are motivated by the lowest human need that is currently unmet. So, for example, when we arrive home from work completely famished, we are likely to look for something eat before we check that everything is as we left it (the unconscious examination we make to ensure we have not been burgled). Once we feel safe, our immediate hunger satisfied to some degree, then we can consider greeting those we live with. For the majority of us, the base of the triangle is solid, in that we have sufficient food, adequate shelter and are relatively free from danger. Therefore, we live for most of our time within the top three sections of the triangle, seeking to satisfy our psychological, spiritual and emotional needs. We move from one section to another, depending on the situation and the need which seems most important at any given time (Hayes, 2000). For example, the need for academic success may override the need for food as completing an assignment is prioritised and hunger pangs ignored.

Consider now the patient and family living with cancer. The very diagnosis brings with it uncertainty, fear and threatens the integrity of both the individual and the family in the widest possible context (Sheldon, 2003). No longer can anything be taken for granted, resulting in a major assault to the stability of every level within the triangle. In health, understanding the hierarchy can assist in understanding individual motivation, but can it help us understand the hidden issues of psychosocial care?

The hierarchy and the patient

From the moment the first symptom is detected, psychologically the individual begins to question who they are and face the 'first intimations of mortality' (Neuberger, 1999). There is the possibility that they are no longer, for example the fit, independent wife, mother, father or husband they were before the symptom appeared. The degree to which this concern reaches the conscious level is directly related to the severity of and importance attached to the symptom. The magnitude of the perceived threat grows in importance as the intensity or number of symptoms increases. Whilst on the surface the person may appear calm, continuing with the routines of their everyday life, their self-esteem is so affected that all thoughts of success and personal growth begin to fade into the background. For the person who has had no warning signs and is diagnosed following routine screening, the threat can experienced as acutely as a severe physical blow (Becker, 2001; Hughes, 1999).

Following diagnosis, a management plan should be devised. Depending on the malignancy, this may involve surgery, chemotherapy or radiotherapy and quite possibly a combination of all three. At best, regular attendance at out patient clinics will be necessary, which in the case of radiotherapy could require daily appointments over several weeks. At worst, surgical treatment may require prolonged hospital stays as an in-patient. Between these two extremes are the short monthly admissions to hospital required for chemotherapy. Whatever the treatment modality, it is likely that the patient will spend considerable time away from their home, their work (if employed) and the routines of their everyday life. These necessary absences begin to isolate the individual who, because of their illness, is now significantly different from their family and friends (Sheldon, 2003). Those closely involved in supporting the patient may also experience some degree of isolation. For example, repeated trips to the hospital may erode into their own time, space and priorities (Becker, 2001). They have become a 'family with cancer' and are therefore fundamentally different from families in which there is no cancer.

This isolation may be increased as the effects of treatment take hold. Visible mutilating surgery can be expected to have a detrimental effect on the way the patient interacts with others and how they, in turn, respond to him or her. Whilst the effects of some types of surgery can be covered up from external scrutiny (for example, mastectomy, stoma formation, etc) and thus may not be obvious to outsiders, the patient's perception of their body will be negatively effected. This may influence their ability to interact with others and accurately perceive the behaviour of those around them. The patient can be further isolated by the side-effects of chemotherapy and radiotherapy, such as hair loss, vomiting and fatigue. As the patient becomes increasingly withdrawn from their social group, the needs for security and a sense of safety take priority (Sheldon, 2003).

But how can the patient ever feel safe when their very life is under threat? Every ache or pain potentially becomes evidence that the disease is progressing or the treatment is not working (Hughes, 1999). For patients who are immuno-compromised as a result of treatment, coming into contact with the common cold virus could be potentially fatal. Fears of 'contracting something' may further isolate the patient, as they become wary of venturing into social situations and visitors are viewed as potential carriers of disease.

It is very common for the patient and family to experience financial worries and as these develop, the sense of security becomes even more threatened. Whilst some people are fortunate to have their income protected if they are off work through sickness, others are not, and many more live on state benefits and retirement pensions. Whilst some benefits are available, mainly the Disability Living and Attendance Allowances, these can often fall short of meeting the family's existing financial commitments and the increased demands resulting from the illness. For example, the costs of the frequent visits to hospital, special diets, increased heating bills and even replacing clothes to accommodate the patients weight loss or occasionally weight gain all have to be met somehow.

As the needs in this section of Maslow's triangle can no longer be met, the patient is faced with meeting the basic physiological needs. But as the disease progresses, even eating and drinking become impossible and so, at the point when the patient can no longer meet any of their needs, death arrives.

It would appear from this description that wherever an individual is in the hierarchy, the diagnosis of cancer sends them spiralling downward, the pace of descent determined by a combination of the type of cancer, its treatment and the resources of the individual and family. The role of the health or social care worker in this scenario is to support the patient in their downward journey. Through effective and sensitive communication, the patient and family can be encouraged to express their psychosocial needs (Kinghorn, 2001), enabling professionals to be proactive in preventing problems and reactive if they should occur. For example, as social isolation develops, we can offer day care; as security becomes increasingly threatened, we can organise benefits and additional support (ie. home care or, if needed, admission to a care home); and when the patient can no longer manage to meet their basic needs, we can wash, feed and toilet them.

Whilst 'the hierarchy of human needs' (Maslow, 1970) offers some insights into the effect of progressive malignant disease for the psychosocial well-being of an individual and family, as it stands it is unhelpful as a framework for understanding the hidden challenges of psychosocial care from the patient's perspective. If, however, the hierarchy is viewed from another perspective, its use becomes clearer.

An alternative perspective

While we are well and free from illness, we strive towards the pinnacle of Maslow's triangle, the point of maximal personal growth and development. But once we become sick, this slips further and further from our grasp. Therefore, consider the effect if we allow the diagnosis of a life-threatening illness to act in some way as a catalyst to turn around the priorities within the hierarchy (*Figure 7.3*). Personal growth and self-fulfilment now become the base that supports all our other needs, and from which we begin our quest to meet them. If we can recognise that our *raison d'être* no longer requires us to strive to climb the hierarchy of needs, we content ourselves in who we are and what we have become — ie. our personal growth and self-fulfilment. Whatever our condition, either as a result of the disease or its treatment, we are still able to experience growth and development, thus increasing our sense of self-fulfilment.

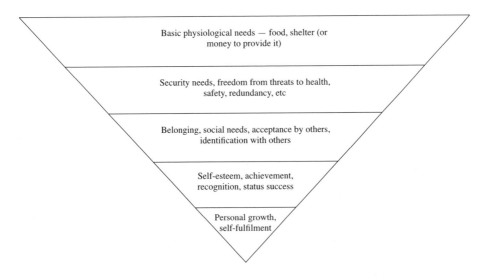

Figure 7.3: Inverted 'triangle of human needs'

Those actions and strategies that emphasise, protect and strengthen this new base therefore address the hidden aspects of psychosocial care. On a practical level, this may involve enabling an individual to achieve some life-long ambition (within the constraints imposed by the patient's physical condition), restore damaged or broken relationships, or complete a personal project. Addressing the hidden aspects of psychosocial care, therefore, involves enabling the patient to recognise all they have achieved throughout their life and indeed are continuing to achieve now. Although goals may be much smaller, they are no less important. A key requirement is to move the emphasis from the past and the future to concentrate in the 'here and now'. For example, in the past the patient may have eaten a three-course meal three times daily, but now, for today, three spoonfuls of soup is sufficient. On retirement, the patient may have planned to travel around the world, but now, for today, walking to the toilet with a walking stick is what can be achieved.

Whilst some patients may be able, unaided, to reconcile past events and relationships in order to make sense of their lives, thus reaching a sense of self-fulfilment, others require help and support to do so. Whilst we cannot ignore the patient's needs for other components of the hierarchy, such as shelter and nutrition, if we are to accept the challenge of psychological care, including it's hidden aspects, we must be prepared to work with them so they increase their sense of fulfilment.

Viewing the hierarchy from this angle provides a useful framework for health and social care professionals when caring for patients' psychosocial needs. Personal growth and fulfilment is no longer viewed as something to be dealt with when all else is finished, but the fundamental basis of all care.

The hierarchy and the family

Family members of a patient with cancer have their own psychosocial needs, which, although related to those of the patients, are unique to them. Indeed, they too have a hierarchy of needs and function on a similar level to the patient pre-diagnosis. With the news of the diagnosis and all that is associated with it, they too receive a severe emotional shock and are besieged with questions relating to who they are and how they will cope (Sheldon, 2003). Like the patient, their security is threatened, their foundations shaken, and their anticipated future lost, creating an uncomfortable emotional burden (Becker, 2001). Unlike the patient, however, the question of their long-term survival is not really in any doubt. Throughout the course of the illness, they will continue to function at different levels of the triangle, albeit moving up and down between sections as circumstances dictate. The overall direction of their journey, however, remains upwards.

Since they themselves do no have a life-threatening disease, their triangle continues to point in the direction that Maslow (1970) intended, whilst that of their loved one is inverted. This may explain the source of the conflict that can occur within the family unit (Becker, 2001). The internal motivators for members of the family are encouraging them to move upwards towards self-fulfilment whilst the patient has already reached that point, irrespective of what their physical condition allows them to do.

To illustrate this point, consider the very basic need for food. We all know that our very survival depends on our ability to eat and drink. As the patient progresses along the cancer journey, the desire to eat decreases. Very few cancer patients, in the later stages of their disease, complain of hunger, and fewer still are bothered by an inability to eat (Finegan, 1999). As the Maslow triangle has become inverted, the need for food is no longer a primary motivator. But for the carers, whose triangle remains upright, it continues to be of utmost importance. For many, the reluctance and often refusal to take specially prepared nutritional offerings is taken as a sign of personal rejection, and an indication that they are no longer needed or valued (Doyle, 1996).

Thus conflict arises, which can be explained by the inversion of the patient's Maslow triangle. For the carers, moving upwards in the triangle is of paramount importance, but for the patient, with an inverted triangle, moving upwards is optional. No matter how close the patient and members of the family are, in sickness as in health they have to move through their respective triangles independently of each other. For the family, this movement is not only necessary, but also an inherent activity of life.

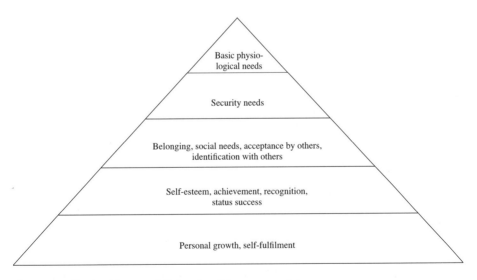

Figure 7.4: Revised inverted 'triangle of human needs'

A final word

Inverting the Maslow triangle, however, results in it balancing on its apex. This leaves it very unstable and likely to topple over with the least disturbance or upset. Perhaps this is a good diagrammatic representation of how the patient feels after diagnosis and throughout treatment. The vast majority of patients, however, are not alone, but supported by friends and family. These supporters bring with them their own upright triangles of needs, which when placed alongside the patient's inverted triangle, provide buffers, helping to keep it upright. We could therefore describe the role of health and social care workers addressing psychosocial needs in palliative care patients as enabling the patient and family to 'keep the triangle balanced'. This could be achieved in working with the patient, the family or indeed both, either together or individually. For the patient without friends and family, the role of the health care workers is to provide the required balance.

But the hidden aspects of psychosocial care require more than this. The aim must be to enable the triangle to stand independently, not merely by providing support, but by enabling a fundamental change in shape (*Figure 7.4*). In achieving this change in shape, the triangle now provides stability and a firm foundation for the patient when all other needs no longer matter.

References

Alexander DA (2001) Psychosocial research in palliative care. In: Doyle D, Hanks GWC, Macdonald N (eds) *The Oxford Textbook of Palliative Medicine*. Oxford: OUP

Becker R (2001) How will I cope?: psychological aspects of advanced illness. In: Kinghorn S, Gamlin R (eds) *Palliative Nursing Bringing Comfort and Hope*. London: Ballière Tindall

Buckman R (2001) Communicating in palliative care: a practical guide. In: Doyle D, Hanks GWC, Macdonald N (eds) *The Oxford Textbook of Palliative Medicine*. Oxford: OUP

Doyle D (1996) *Domicillary Palliative Care: a Guide for the Primary Care Team*. Oxford: OUP

Finegan W (1999) *Helpful Essential Links to Palliative Care*. London: Macmillan Cancer Relief

Gross RD (2001) *Psychology — the Science of Mind and Behaviour*. 4th edition. London: Edward Arnold

Hayes N (2000) *Foundations of Psychology*. London: Thompson Learning

Hockley J (1997) The evolution of the hospice approach. In: Clark D, Hockley J, Ahmedzai S (eds) *New Themes in Palliative Care*. Buckingham: Open University Press

Hughes J (1999) *Cancer and Emotion: a Practical Guide to Psycho-oncology*. Chichester: John Wiley & Sons

Jeffrey D (2003) What do we mean by psychosocial care in palliative care? In: Lloyd-Williams M (ed) *Psychosocial Issues in Palliative Care*. Oxford: OUP

Johnson J (1998) The notion of spiritual care in practice. In: Cobb M, Robshaw V (eds) *The Spiritual Challenge of Health Care*. London: Churchill Livingstone

Kinghorn S (2001) Communication in advanced illness: challenges and opportunities. In: Kinghorn S, Gamlin R (eds) *Palliative Nursing Bringing Comfort and Hope*. London: Ballière Tindall

Lugton J (1999) Support processes in palliative care. In: Lugton J, Kindlen M (eds) *Palliative Care: The Nursing Role*. Edinburgh: Churchill Livingston

Lugton J (2002) *Communicating with Dying People and their Relatives*. Abingdon: Radcliffe Medical Press

Marson S, Hartlebury M, Johnston R, Scammell B (1992) Managing People. Basingstoke: Macmillan

Maslow A (1970) *Motivation and Personality*. New York: Harper & Row

McIntyre R (1999) Support for family and carers. In: Lugton J, Kindlen M (eds) *Palliative Care: The Nursing Role*. Edinburgh: Churchill Livingston

NICE (2004) *Guidance on Cancer Services: Improving Supportive and Palliative Care for Adults with Cancer*. London: NICE

NCHSPCS (1997) *Feeling Better: Psychosocial Care in Specialist Palliative Care*. London: NCHSPCS

Neuberger J (1999) Dying Well: A Guide to Enabling a Good Death. Cheshire: Hochland & Hochland

Parkes CM (1971) Psychological transitions: a field for study. *Soc Sci Med* **5**: 101–15

Saunders C (1958) Dying of cancer. *St Thomas's Hospital Gazette* **56**(2): 37–47

Sheldon F (1997) *Psychosocial Palliative Care: Good Practice in the Care of the Dying and Bereaved*. Cheltenham: Stanley Thornes

Sheldon F (2003) Social impact of advanced cancer. In: Lloyd-Williams M (ed) *Psychosocial Issues in Palliative Care*. Oxford: OUP

Sutherland N, Gamlin R (1999) Body image and sexuality: implications for palliative care. In: Lugton J, Kindlen M (eds) *Palliative Care: The Nursing Role*. Edinburgh: Churchill Livingston

Thompson D (1995) (ed) *The Concise Oxford Dictionary of Current English*. Oxford: Claredon Press

Walker L, Walker M, Sharp D (2003) Current provision of psychosocial care within palliative care. In: Lloyd-Williams M (ed) *Psychosocial Issues in Palliative Care*. Oxford: OUP

8

Spirituality and palliative care

Wilf McSherry

Introduction

It can be taken for granted that healthcare professionals acknowledge that the concept of spirituality has a fundamental and central role to play within the provision of health care. This is evident in the vast amount of books, articles, and research studies published on the subject. In recent years, this interest has escalated, resulting in a proliferation of available material (including websites), with annual conferences and study days being held on spirituality in the context of palliative care. Increasingly, the deliberations on 'spirituality' have changed. Rather than the concept being debated and investigated purely theoretically, adopting a 'universal' or 'global' approach, the emphasis is now on examining and developing the 'pragmatics' (practical relevance and applications) for different spheres of practice. What seems to be occurring is a realisation of the importance of spirituality, however defined, within the context of peoples' lives. Specialist areas are now seeking to take ownership, applying the concept of spirituality at 'grass roots' level. This has resulted in most of the Allied Health Professions (AHP) engaging and grappling with the 'thorny' concept (Swinton and Narayanasmay, 2002).

The area of palliative care has not escaped or been immune to this changing agenda. Indeed, if one believes what has been written on the subject from within palliative care, then it would be fair to assume that the provision of spiritual care is imperative if practitioners are to maintain an individual's sense of well-being when living with any form of life-threatening or life-limiting illness. This chapter explores what is meant by the term 'spirituality' and 'spiritual care'. The title of this chapter, 'Spirituality and palliative care', implies that they are two distinct and separate concepts. However, it will be shown that spirituality has a fundamental and central (often hidden) role to play within the context of palliative care in that we cannot have one without the other. The chapter will explore some important theoretical and practical debates that are affecting the way that spirituality is managed within the context of palliative care.

Contextualising spirituality

Throughout the last decade, several documents and directives have been published that seek to shape the delivery of palliative care (World Health Organisation [WHO], 1990; Calman and Hine, 1995; National Council for Hospice and Specialist Palliative Care Services, 1997; Department of Health [DoH], 2000; National Institute for Clinical Excellence, 2004). These publications appear to emphasis the importance of practitioners in all areas of 'health care' being informed and implementing key principles in the provision of effective palliative care, highlighting the importance of 'recognizing and managing spiritual problems' (Carroll, 2001). The idea that all patients and staff should receive support with spiritual matters is clearly stated in the NICE (2004) guidance on cancer services. This document contains an entire section (seven) entitled 'Spiritual Support Services'. The fact that this section is included is a step towards formalising and operationalising spiritual care, thereby affirming the importance of this dimension of palliative care. In the past, it was often thought that palliative care equated only with 'hospice care' and that individuals with any form of life-threatening illness (predominantly cancer) should receive 'specialist' intervention from 'specialist practitioners' and that palliative care could not be effectively managed within 'general' care settings by 'general staff'.

One cannot deny the benefits to be gained through receiving care from 'specialists' or 'palliative care teams' who possess expert knowledge and skills in the managements of certain diseases or symptoms (Moss, 2002). However, it would be naïve to think that since the implementation of the above policies and standards, the provision of palliative care is now effectively managed in all primary or secondary care settings. The provision of effective palliative care that is equitable and accessible by all is still not a reality. It is important to highlight that the concept of spirituality is either implicit (hidden) or explicit within the desire to provide effective and efficient palliative care.

Hidden aspects

Taylor (2003) clearly articulates the hidden aspects of spirituality: 'Patients wish that nurses provide kindness, connectedness, prayerfulness, physical support, and so forth.' This list suggests that the provision of spiritual care need not be something extra that is brought into palliative care. Many healthcare professionals will be displaying these qualities not under the proviso of 'spirituality'. Instead, by fulfilling their daily roles and responsibilities delivering essential care to patients and their families, they are attending to the spiritual dimension. Healthcare professionals (and, it must be added, volunteers) working in palliative care services may not be overtly aware or articulate 'I'm meeting my patient's spiritual needs' but they are already delivering spiritual care' and successfully meeting the spiritual needs of their patients in a covert manner. Byrne (2002) writes:

> *It could be said that nurses are involved with spiritual care without necessarily being conscious of having the language to articulate the nature of the experience.*

This raises the issue that perhaps the concept of spirituality and the provision of 'spiritual care' have remained hidden because they are conveyed and communicated under another vocabulary — perhaps that of loss, grief, fear, and 'holism' (Draper and McSherry, 2002). This is a language with which many healthcare professionals are familiar and, it must be stressed, comfortable.

Philosophical orientation

If one explores the aforementioned documents and traces the inception of the 'hospice movement', it is instantly recognisable that one of the predominant features of specialist palliative care services is a commitment (Byrne, 2002; Walter, 2002) to the philosophy of 'holism' or 'holistic care'. This commitment has subsequently been transferred to the development of specialist palliative care service. This 'written' commitment is evident in the DoH's *The NHS Cancer Plan* (2000), which states: 'The principles of palliative care — holistic, patient-centred care — apply across all conditions and in all settings.' The plan could have gone further and actually used the word 'spirituality' or made reference to the spiritual dimension within their definition of holism, thus raising the profile and importance of spirituality within this agenda. Furthermore, initiatives and future developments seem to be focused more on medical, physiological and organisational improvements, with only fleeting mention of other fundamental issues related to psychosocial or spiritual well-being. It would seem that spirituality is 'implicitly' not 'explicitly' mentioned; that there is inference rather than direct reference. But perhaps politicians and bureaucrats, through the lack of direct reference, 'unknowingly' preserve the integrity of spirituality because it is not isolated — that is, not raised as another objective to be met.

Hawkett (1998) makes direct reference to the importance of spirituality within the context of palliative care when she writes:

> *We all recognised — and had a desire to respond to — the spiritual needs of those facing death, but we lacked a common approach. We*

realised that as the subject had aroused such passion and diversity, spirituality in the palliative care context was worthy of a whole issue of IJPN.

Hawkett stresses the ambiguity, diversity and subjectivity surrounding the area of spirituality, underlining and affirming the place spirituality has within peoples' lives, and acknowledging and endorsing activity associated with this dimension of palliative care.

Defining 'holism'

'Holism' can be defined as recognition that all dimensions of the individual, physical, social, psychological and spiritual are attended to with equal importance (McSherry, 2000a). 'The whole is greater than its constituent parts' is one phrase often used to describe holism (Bradshaw, 1994). If one subscribes to this view, then holism is about looking at the entire individual, because 'all dimensions' means 'the whole person'. It is not about fragmenting or reducing individuals into manageable units, but appreciating how all the units of the person may be interconnected and interact with each other.

This 'whole' approach to holism is not often reinforced in health care. Instead, the terms 'holistic care' or 'total patient care' are often used. 'Holism' is often depicted diagrammatically as a circle or square divided into quarters. This approach to holism is still reductionist because the person is divided into manageable units (for example, the quarters are often physical, social, psychological, with the spiritual tagged on at the end as an afterthought). Sadly, this approach to holism is still evident in contemporary palliative care.

However, this segmental or reductionist model does not emphasises how all dimensions of the person are integrated and dependant on each other in order to maintain a sense of physical, psychological, social and spiritual well-being or state of harmony. The hidden danger for palliative care is that if we 'fragment' or detach spirituality from the heart of holistic care, it may just be seen as another area to address. Elsdon (1995) highlights the integrating and unifying force of spirituality within the context of peoples' lives, asserting that, as an individual's physical health declines, greater emphasis and importance may be placed on the spiritual dimension.

Bradshaw's (1994) concern is that if 'spirituality' is isolated and viewed out of context — that is, set aside and viewed in isolation as an area for attention or study — then it may become disengaged. Then, rather than providing 'integrated care', individuals are fragmented and the spiritual dimension becomes another category or box to be ticked, another aspect of care to be attended. The net effect may be that there is a dislocation of the spiritual, a loss of integrity in that the individual is no longer viewed as a 'whole' but as a discrete set of manageable mechanistic units.

From this brief analysis of holism, the exact and precise nature of spirituality and how it operates and resides within peoples' lives are very mysterious and subjective issues. The precise nature of this relationship will possibly be the source of many debates for years to come. However, palliative care cannot be delivered in a holistic manner if spirituality is removed from the notion of holism, either in the sense that it does not appear there in the first place, or it is 'fragmented out' and seen purely as a separate entity. Spirituality is the thread or force that penetrates, integrates and harmonises all dimensions of a person in an equal, unique, hidden and mysterious manner.

Defining 'spirituality'

There is no real authoritative (Narayanasmay, 2001) or definitive definition of spirituality. Hunt *et al* (2003) indicate that, potentially, people may have diverse orientations or views of spirituality that are dependent on their own world view. For some individuals, their spirituality may be shaped and expressed through a formal religious structure, while for other people their spiritual orientation may be fashioned and influenced not by any religious principles, but by humanistic or secular beliefs, the descriptors or defining characteristics of which could be highly varied (Wright, 2002; McSherry and Cash, 2004).

Refining the concepts and theories

McEwen and Wills (2002) suggest that concepts and theories are representations of an individual's thoughts, ideas and views of a given phenomenon. Needless to say, these may be very subjective and open to interpretation. It is refreshing to see that the conceptual and theoretical arguments shrouding spirituality are now coming under some scrutiny and investigation. Indeed, some of these debates are originating in and being focused on palliative care (Byrne, 2002; Walter, 2002). These debates are heartening and refreshing because rather than ideas surrounding spirituality being cyclical (refashioned, repackaged and continually recapitulated), people are now starting to consider the implications and consequences of the concepts, theories and discourse presented. This refocusing will help to develop and refine the language of spirituality and will ultimately lead to its greater application to practice.

Before exploring some of these concerns, it may be useful to provide some definitions of spirituality that have been formulated within palliative care and nursing circles.

Various definitions of spirituality

The literature surrounding spirituality reveals that the concept is shrouded in subjectivity and ambiguity. An individual's spirituality seems to be shaped and influenced by many factors, especially socialisation. Cawley (1998) identifies culture, background, upbringing and social contexts as having significant influence on the development of an individual's spirituality. If one accepts these influences, it would seem that spirituality might be defined in various ways. One argument put forward is that spiritual formation is dependent on an individual's own philosophy or world-view (Martsolf and Mickley, 1998). While there is a need to acknowledge the individualistic nature of spirituality, we must not loose sight of the other global or communal influences that may unconsciously have fashioned the individual through parenting, institutions and cultural influences. This point may be significant when undertaking life review or a spiritual history because such force may have had a positive or negative effect, the ramifications of which can be long-lasting and profound.

A review of some of the definitions of spirituality in palliative and nursing care suggests that spirituality is an eclectic (Cobb, 2001) or a catch-all phrase encompassing a wide range of defining characteristics (*Box 8.1*). These definitions reveal that spirituality has many defining attributes and hidden layers of meaning. The complex and mysterious elements of life are entwined and intermingled. The net effect is that spirituality can take on many forms or guises. Spirituality will be experienced and expressed differently by different individuals. The definitions outlined (*Box 8.1*) reveal that spirituality may accommodate a wide range of theological, philosophical, sociological, even environments factors. Many of these factors and forces are hidden, and their influence on the individual very powerful. For some individuals, spirituality may be that which gives their life meaning and purpose; for others it may be the adherence to a particular belief system that gives structure and direction. Finally, spirituality may be based upon superstition or myth. The net effect is that spirituality is not something that can be simply explained; neither is it easily articulated, since the language and expression may not be able to convey the full extent of what one believes, and why.

This is very important when addressing the subject within the context of palliative care. Providers of health care must guard against assumption and generalisation with regard to what constitutes 'spirituality'. This note of caution is urged because some individuals, patients and healthcare professionals will not readily identify with the definitions, language, descriptors and metaphors used in health care.

Box 8.1: Definitions of spirituality

A quality that goes beyond religious affiliation, that strives for inspirations, reverence, awe, meaning and purpose, even in those who do not believe in any good. The spiritual dimension tries to be in harmony with the universe, and strives for answers about the infinite, and comes into focus when the person faces emotional stress, physical illness or death.

Murray and Zentner (1989)

The spiritual realm can be broadly defined as the life force springing from the unknown that pervades each person's entire being. It encompasses the volitional, emotional, ethical, social, intellectual and physical dimensions. It is the centre or core that integrates the whole person, surpassing the biological and the psychosocial. It is the self, or I, the essence of personhood, the God within, that which communicates with the transcendent. It is the part of each individual that aspires to ultimate awareness, meaning, value, purpose, beauty, dignity, relatedness and integrity. The spiritual is the source of faith, hope and courage. It inspires theology, artistic inspiration and expression, love and healing.

O'Rawe Amenta (1998)

Spirituality is a personal search for meaning and purpose in life, which may or may not be related to religion. It entails connection to self-chosen and or religious beliefs, values and practices that give meaning to life, thereby inspiring and motivating individuals to achieve their optimal being. This connection brings faith, hope, peace, and empowerment. The results are joy, forgiveness of oneself and others, awareness and acceptance of hardship and mortality, a heightened sense of physical and emotional well-being, and the ability to transcend beyond the infirmities of existence.

Tanyi (2002)

Categorisation and discourse

Cawley's (1998) exploration of the concept of spirituality highlighted that spirituality can be explained in two broad categorises — the first, relating to religious connotations, and the second to non-religious connotations. More recently, Rumbold (2002) has suggested that there are four strands emerging with regard to approaches to spiritual care:

- identity
- meaning
- alliances
- alternative spiritual belief.

'Identity' is normally expressed and created when the individual is able to answer the question 'Who am I?' 'Meaning' concerns that element of life that provides an individual with a sense of meaning and purpose, from which fulfilment comes. 'Alliances' refers to the people and partnerships created that an individual may develop through adherence to a particular framework (religious), from which one derives hope. 'Alternative spiritual belief' is similar to the above but involves beliefs that lie outside any religious sphere.

Rumbold argues that these four strands may be complementary within the individual. He suggests that an understanding of these strands is important because they may influence healthcare interest and future direction with regards to the provision of spiritual care. A disruption in any of these strands may result in the individual experiencing a spiritual need, perhaps expressed as a loss of identify, a search for meaning, or the re-evaluation of one's involvement within a particular belief, institution or community, whether religious or secular. Closer analysis of Cawley's and Rumbold's categorisations confirms that much of the debate surrounding spirituality still falls into two broad classifications: believers and none-believers. Or, what Bash (2004) terms the 'the non-theistic approach', 'the theistic approach' and 'the via media'.

Believers and non-believers

The definitions presented (*Box 8.1*) suggest that many working within health care take it for granted that spirituality is a universal phenomenon. Puchalski and Romer (2000), providing general recommendations for clinicians undertaking a spiritual assessment, state: 'Consider spirituality as a potentially important component of every patient's physical well-being and mental health'. For many individuals, spirituality is shaped, moulded and directly influenced by formal religious beliefs and practices. Traditionally, spirituality and religion were viewed as synonymous (religion, in this context, being the adherence to a set of prescribed beliefs, rituals and practices that provide the individual with a pattern or 'blueprint' for living). This association persists today, and many people are unable to perceive spirituality as anything other than belief in a 'religion'. However, within health care, this approach to spirituality has been challenged and the concept of spirituality has been extended to include 'everyone', even those who do not believe in any God or practice any formal religion. The reason for drawing attention to these two distinct groups will become clearer. To highlight the different approaches to spirituality, some excerpts from interview transcripts will be used. The data were obtained from an ongoing qualitative study that I am currently undertaking. An overview of the research study is provided (*Box 8.2*)

Box 8.2: Overview of study

Method — qualitative grounded theory

Data collection — interviews were done between March 2001 and July 2003

Participants — nursing (twenty-four people), chaplaincy (seven), social work (one), occupational therapy (one), physiotherapy (two), patients (fourteen), public (four)

Sex — male (twenty-four), female (twenty-nine)

Religions — Christianity (twenty-seven), Islam (two), Hinduism (one), Sikhism (one), Judaism (one)

Location — Area I = hospice, areas II & III = Large Acute Trust

Analysis — Constant comparative analysis

Patients' perspectives

Having spoken to fourteen patients about their perceptions of spirituality, what appears to be emerging is a polarisation of opinion. On the far left, there are patients, users and many groups within the 'general public' with what could be categorised as a conservative, traditional understanding of spirituality, possibly representing the general public's discourse. For these patients, their general understanding is spirituality 'equals' religion. McSherry and Cash (2004) suggest that there is a 'traditional' form of spirituality that derives its meaning and language from religious traditions. Bradshaw (1994) and Pattison (2001) argue strongly that once spirituality is removed from its religious context and discourse, it is in danger of becoming meaningless. There is a growing unease within healthcare circles that there is a drive to divorce or even remove the theist and the religious from spirituality. However, this does not seem to be deliberate but reflects a desire to achieve universal inclusion and application of spirituality, both at an individual and community level.

The 'traditional' understanding described is evident in the excerpts of conversation provided, where four patients who were living with a life-threatening illness or approaching death were asked (by me) about their understanding of the term 'spirituality' (*Box 8.3*).

Box 8.3: Patients' perceptions of spirituality

Respondent one

Well that's what I thought when I got this letter, you know. Well, I thought, well again we're back to religion! You know I'm Church of England!

Respondent two

Well, from national service days I was the only one in the British army with two religions in the pay book. And I had two religions for the simple reason is, if it was fall out RC's [Roman Catholic] I used to fall out and go do something else. And if it was fall out C of E's [Church of England], I used to go and fall out [laughing] and they caught up with me in the finish. But say it has never interested me.

Respondent three

I think everyone has spirituality but the majority of us have it at very low level. I think it goes back to almost oestolapithesis, when man stood upright. This is noticeable in a photograph of a man and a woman walking over pumice and a child following jumping in their parents' footsteps. You can see it on the beach now. That was just a hint that man was becoming human. I think it was built in strongly to early man almost as a warning signal or a defence signal. He knew or he could sense when he was in danger, everyone wanted a bite out of him! And it was this extra sense. It has now been knocked out of us. Our brains are crammed full of rubbish — TV, letters, and information.

Respondent four

Well, I'm not religious at all!

It must be stressed that not all the patients shared the same visions or perspective; on the contrary, some offered elaborate and articulate definitions (Respondent Three) that mirrored those of the nurses. Similarly, some patients felt that spirituality was associated with ghosts, ghouls, 'spiritualism' and attending séances to contact the dead. These traditional approaches to understanding spirituality did not seem to be shared by many of the allied health professions represented in this study. These individuals were able to describe and articulate broad and detailed descriptions of spirituality, some of which could be categorised as 'postmodern' in thinking.

Having explained the far left (traditional) perception of spirituality, there is a need to provide some explanation as to what constitutes the 'far right' or postmodern perspective. This has been categorised as the new spirituality, couched in terms of new age and free thinking.

Healthcare professionals' perspectives

Speaking to thirty-five people from most of the allied health professions revealed that many of them had a broad understanding of spirituality (*Box 8.4*). The four definitions provided illustrate that for them, spirituality is a universal phenomena, residing in all people, believers and unbelievers. This is in stark contrast to the patients' interviewed, who were unable to distinguish spirituality from religion.

Box 8.4: Healthcare professionals' perceptions of spirituality

Nurse

I think it's what makes the person, the person they are, you know, their personality, how they think, how they behave and it affects, just affects an individual, in every way really. I don't think you can say right today I'm going to be spiritual, I don't think you can do that. I just think it's how you are and what person you are.

Social worker

I certainly don't see spirituality as belonging to a religion; I don't see it as that. And I think that probably because I don't have a practising faith at the moment. Working at the hospice and seeing people die and it just makes me doubt the existence of a forgiving merciful God. So I can't see it, doesn't fit comfortably spirituality and religion to me. The chaplain and I have lots of interesting conversations and discussions, which he always wins. Because he's got lots of information and experience from the religious point of view! So you come away from these conversations feeling very dissatisfied. So it's certainly not there! It sort of experiences I think to me, things that things that you know I find meaningful, think awe the wow factor!

Physiotherapist

I knew it was about finding meaning in life, whatever that might be, feeling a sense of purpose, and almost like that for me life is about finding a sense of purpose and meaning and doing what feels right, what feels your life purpose or path. For me, if I've been doing that, then my life feels more comfortable, if I've been fighting against it then it's not!

> **Box 8.4 continued...**
>
> **Chaplain**
>
> My current understanding is that it's three-fold. The meaning-purpose aspect, which is most often talked about, is only part of spirituality, and I would say that equally at least relationships and I still struggle to find the right word. A sense of transcendence, awe, wonder, mystery are also important parts of spirituality and spiritual care.

Emerging dichotomy

The dilemma for palliative care is that a dichotomy is emerging over what constitutes 'spirituality'. The implication of this dichotomy is that if this area is not managed sensitively within palliative care, there may well be the potential to alienate a large portion of the people from this debate — namely, patients. Furthermore, the routine use and introduction of spiritual assessment tools and the general acceptance that 'everyone' understands what is meant by the word 'spirituality' may need to be reconsidered (Markham, 1998; McSherry and Ross, 2002). The preliminary findings of this research reveal that there are different ways of perceiving and approaching spirituality, some of which may be professionally or culturally determined. The implications of these diverse perceptions may have an impact on the way that spiritual issues are addressed and managed within the context of palliative care.

Spiritual issues within the context of palliative care

The previous section explored some of the diverse language, myths and definitions of spirituality. The conclusion reached was that academic discourse is not really helpful when trying to transfer such rhetoric into practice. Indeed, several authors (Oldnall, 1996; Nolan and Crawford, 1997) have argued that the theoretical talk surrounding spirituality is unhelpful, and may need to be refined so that the language and metaphors surrounding spirituality are recognised by, and reflect the voices of, practitioners. This is necessary for all areas of healthcare practice, but possibly more so in the area of palliative care. With regard to palliative care, three fundamental debates seem to be emerging that may ultimately shape and direct the way that spiritual care is provided within the specialty (*Box 8.5*).

Box 8.5: Emerging debates

❖ Skills development

❖ Psychological versus spiritual? — or a case of integrated care?

❖ Education

Skills development

Walters (2002) draws attention to a very important point in relation to the provision of spiritual care: that this dimension of care may be an opportunity for some staff while it could be perceived as a burden for others. Walter subscribes to the arguments surrounding the different language and meanings associated with spirituality, since not all people will share the same understanding of spirituality. Therefore, some patients and healthcare professionals working within palliative care services may not be able to accompany or assist patients all the way along their life journey for cultural, religious or personal reasons. The realisation that healthcare professionals must meet the spiritual needs of all their patients must be amended, and this may relieve some of the burden felt by staff in this area. Walter's approach reinforces the individuality of patients and staff and the perception that spiritual care is not just for a select few, but must involve the 'whole team'.

The provision of spiritual care, therefore, may be both threatening and challenging — threatening in the sense that if this area of practice is not undertaken sensitively, there is the potential for patients and practitioners to feel uncomfortable and out of their depth; and challenging because this will undoubtedly require practitioners and patients to engage with issues that may have been extremely painful, often without any immediate resolution. These types of situation often necessitate the need for the patient and practitioner to learn from each other, thereby raising the spectre of vulnerability. However, this is not to say that the provision of spiritual care is all doom and gloom. On the contrary: effective spiritual care is about coming alongside the patient in both the good and bad events of life, and sharing in the joy and sadness. This picture is not one of professional dominance, but of a partnership where mutual trust and respect are shared and fostered.

Taylor *et al* (1994) recognise the inherent dangers in the scientific, medical model where spiritual care is perceived as 'something given by a nurse to a care recipient'. The inevitable pitfall for palliative care, if it were to adopt this model, is the institution of a very didactic, prescriptive pedagogy that perpetuates the medical model of dependence — that is, the healthcare professional is in a position of authority and power, giving care to those in need: the powerless (Mayer, 1992).

Medicalisation and bureaucratisation

Turner (1996) proposes that the area of palliative care has not been immune to the 'negative influences' of medicalisation, with a growing emphasis being placed on describing, measuring and quantifying actions. Turner argues that within the context of palliative care, practitioners appear to be 'doing more' in terms of bureaucratisation, which means they may be caring less for patients. The emphasis within palliative care appears to have changed, and the value of 'presence' and being with patients has been devalued and replaced with 'outcomes', 'measures' and 'targets'. It could be argued that palliative care needs to regain, rediscover and reinvest in those founding principles, where the scientific and spiritual dimensions were inextricable. The over-emphasis on the scientific and bureaucratic agendas seem to have led to the introduction of such things as spiritual-care standards and spiritual assessment tools, without giving due consideration to the ramifications for patients or practitioners.

Assessment of spiritual need

Within palliative care and health care generally (McSherry and Ross, 2002), there is a growing unease with the area of spiritual assessment. Rumbold (2002) writes:

> *Thus we need to reject attempts to capture spirituality in a professional discourse (through objective assessment, imposed terminology, etc), while supporting and facilitating patients' own spiritual awareness and the actions and language that express this awareness.*

This quotation confirms the suspicion that health care has created a 'professional discourse' surrounding spirituality that consists of its own language, terminology and meanings. This discourse, as Rumbold (2002) rightly indicates, may not incorporate or indeed reflect the views, perceptions and life stories of patients living with a life-threatening illness, or facing death. This then raises the question — do we need spiritual assessment? Several authors have offered suggestions for undertaking such an activity (Dudley *et al*, 1995; Muncy, 1996; Puchalski and Romer, 2000). Probably the most pioneering and seminal work is that developed by Ruth Stoll (1979) who presented 'guidelines for spiritual assessment'. It would appear that many tools used within palliative care contexts are derivatives or modifications of this approach.

While spiritual assessment tools draw attention to the spiritual dimension, they must not replace other skills already possessed and used by healthcare professionals and volunteers working within palliative care, such as interpersonal and observation skills. The dangers with introducing any form of assessment tool are that they can be perceived as 'once-only' instruments to be performed on admission. This type of approach does not acknowledge that individuals may not present or declare any spiritual need at first contact, since no rapport or trusting relationship has been formed to facilitate possible disclosure. Further, by using spiritual assessment tools, there are three further assumptions made: first, that all patients have spiritual needs; second, that patients will understand the language; and, third, that the assessing practitioner feels comfortable using the assessment tool and, possibly more importantly, that they have the requisite skills to support the patient should a spiritual need be identified.

Frameworks for education and practice

Many of the assessment tools are usually used in conjunction with a framework for care delivery or education. Within health care (it must be added, predominately nursing), several frameworks have been developed that may assist practitioners in addressing this aspect of care within their practice and education (*Box 8.6*).The majority of these frameworks use a problem-solving or a systematic and cyclical approach to the provision of spiritual care: that is, there are discrete stages that need to be followed, usually starting with assessment, which may then result in planning and formulating a package of care that is implemented with the patient, ending in evaluation. The emphasis on these frameworks is the notion of individualised, patient-centred care. The benefit of using such frameworks is that spirituality may be couched in terms or a language that will be recognisable by patients. More importantly, they will assist in engaging in a dialogue that is culturally sensitive. Simply to ask patients, 'Do you have any spiritual needs?' may be met with a wall of silence or a monosyllabic closed response along the lines of 'C of E' or 'I don't go in for any of that religious stuff.' These frameworks may assist in developing awareness in the spiritual dimension, but the danger is that of fragmentation and duplication of assessment. What is not clear or addressed within these frameworks is the relationship between spiritual and psychological care. These concerns could be extended further to include the physical, psychological and social domains.

Box 8.6: Frameworks for spiritual assessment, spiritual care and education

Govier (2000) — five 'Rs' of spirituality:

- reason
- reflection
- religion
- relationships
- restoration

Ross (1996), McSherry (2000a) — systematic-cyclical approach, incorporating the five phases:

- assessment
- planning
- implementation
- evaluation
- reassessment

Narayanasamy (1999, 2001) — ASSET model:

- actioning spirituality and spiritual care education and training in nursing

Puchalski and Romer (2002) — FICA:

- F: faith or beliefs
- I: importance and influence
- C: community
- A: address

Psychological versus spiritual? Or a case of integrated care?

The National Council for Hospice and Specialist Palliative Care Services (NCHSPCS) (1997) does not define spirituality, making reference only to 'spiritual care':

> *Spiritual care is less tangible and encompasses the emotional benefits of informal support from relatives and friends, participation in religious or other groups, and more formal pastoral care. Many patients feel an increased or renewed need for their religious beliefs and the involvement of an appropriate religious leader is often important.*

This is a narrow definition of spiritual care, and provides a useful contrast to the definitions of spirituality outlined earlier. The main focus of this definition emphasises the religious, pastoral elements, acknowledging the role and support offered by other informal networks. However, there is little or no mention of spiritual care applying to the non-believer — for example, atheists, agnostics and secular humanists, who may be threatened by religiosity (Burnard, 1988). This definition does not seem to accommodate or respond to some of the concerns surrounding the meaning, language and discourse of spirituality. The NCHSPCS (1997) offers the following definition of psychosocial care:

> *Psychosocial care includes psychological approaches concerned with enabling the patient and those close to them to express thoughts, feelings and concerns relating to illness, assessing their individual needs and resources and ensuring that psychological and emotional support is available.*

This quotation suggests psychosocial care uses an interaction model, highlighting specific functions that can be initiated to support patients or those close to them who might express a need in this dimension. In this definition, it would seem that psychosocial care is concerned with allowing individuals to express those thoughts or feelings that may be causing emotional disturbance or anxiety. Psychosocial care is concerned with establishing a confidential, safe and secure environment in which the professional can address such needs. The terminology used in this definition is very similar to that used within the definition of spirituality offered by Murray and Zentner (1989). This presents a further dichotomy and possibly a dilemma for practitioners: how do we distinguish between spiritual need and psychosocial need?

Piles (1990) proposes that there is a need for differentiation of these two important dimensions if the spiritual needs of patients are to be addressed. This is feasible in theory, but perhaps not so easy in practice. Piles (1990) states:

The spiritual dimension is different from the psychosocial dimension in that the former concerns a person's relationship to a higher being or God, as defined by the individual, and the latter concerns itself with the relationship of a person to himself or the environment.

This quotation, rather than clarifying the situation, adds to the confusion. It implies that spirituality is only concerned and distinguishable by a 'theistic' or a transcendent belief, while the psychological is associated with individuality or an 'interconnectedness' with the environment. This approach to the spiritual and psychological domains echoes the views of the NCHSPCS. There is a clear attempt to locate the spiritual within a religious or theistic context, and the psychological is viewed in terms of 'worldly' relationships. These attempts to distinguish, differentiate and ultimately separate do not accommodate the view that spirituality, rather than been something that can be isolated, should be seen as something that permeates and penetrates all aspect of the person.

Perhaps a resolution to this polarisation is to accept that spiritual needs may be manifested (just like psychological needs) through a variety of emotions, feelings and symptoms. So long as these symptoms are managed and the route of the problem(s) or need(s) identified, then should it matter whether the label given is spiritual or psychological? Rather than adopting a simply 'reductionist' model, seeing the physical, psychosocial and spiritual dimensions as separate domains, there is a need to appreciate that all are interconnected and can influence each other in a mysterious manner. At present, the blurring of boundaries and uncertainties associated with these two important dimensions will not be resolved through engaging in purely academic debates.

Education

One of the dilemmas that persists and continues to plague health care, and which is equally relevant to the provision of palliative care, is: how do we prepare practitioners to meet the spiritual needs of their patients? In light of the questions and areas highlighted in this chapter, a further question may be asked: should we educate? There is a growing debate within nursing about educational preparedness to meet the spiritual needs of patients (Narayanasamy, 1993; McSherry and Draper, 1996; Ross, 1996; Bradshaw, 1997; McSherry, 2002b). The central arguments revolve around two educational principles: pedagogy and andragogy. In other words, can the skills required to address the spiritual dimension be taught through formal educational methods? Or is spiritual awareness 'caught' — that is, developed through immersion in clinical practice and being exposed to and sensitised to the needs of individuals in this area? While these debates rumble on, there is a noticeable gap — or, more precisely, a chasm — emerging between the theory generated in the corridors of academia and its applicability and relevance to practice (Oldnall, 1996).

The concerns that a theory-practice gap exists with regard to provision of spiritual care is of fundamental concern. Despite all the academic and professional discourses and achievements that attempt to extricate, elucidate and ultimately define spirituality, the gap between theory and practice continues to grow. Perhaps the main reason for this is that the discourses created by academics are not easily transferable into practice. Further, the language created does not seem to incorporate the voices of patients, service users and practitioners with regard to what they feel their needs and perceptions are in relation to the provision of spiritual care, and how this relates to other essential elements of care. These shortcomings must be addressed if the spiritual dimension is to be better understood and managed within the context of palliative care.

Conclusion

This chapter has explored the part that spirituality plays in palliative care. Several fundamental debates have been raised in relation to the language and discourses that have been developed within health care. It seems that the time is now right for academics and all members of the palliative care team to revisit and re-engage with some of the 'thorny' issues associated with spirituality. If this activity is not undertaken with some haste, there is an inherent danger that the concept of spirituality and the 'diverse spiritualities' being promulgated may have no relevance to service users. The hidden meanings associated with spirituality need to be refined so that they truly reflect and represent the perceptions of those whom palliative care is asked to serve.

The conceptual and theoretical arguments that have been constructed around spirituality seem to have isolated and fragmented this dimension of care. If palliative care continues down this route, then spirituality, rather than being an integrating force, will be seen as another area to be addressed, with the risk of turning it into another managerial, organisational chore. The realisation that many professionals and volunteers within palliative care may be already attending to and effectively meeting their patients' spiritual needs requires consideration. Will raising the conscious awareness of patients and healthcare professionals with regard to 'spirituality' and 'spiritual care' bring clarification? Or will it exacerbate the confusion and ambiguity that already exist?

Perhaps a resolution to these questions and debates may be found in an appreciation and acceptance that the provision of spiritual care is not about isolation and fragmentation, but a realisation that this dimension is often hidden beyond language, and thereby integrated within the care that is already provided in a palliative setting.

References

Amenta MO (1997) Spiritual care: the heart of palliative nursing. *Int J Palliat Nurs* **3**(1): 4

Bash A (2004) Spirituality: the emperor's new clothes? *J Clin Nurs* **13**: 11–16

Bradshaw A (1994) *Lighting the Lamp: the Spiritual Dimension of Nursing Care.* London: Scutaria Press

Bradshaw A (1997) Teaching spiritual care to nurses: an alternative approach. *Int J Palliat Nurs* **3**(1): 51–7

Burnard P (1988) The spiritual needs of atheists and agnostics. *Prof Nurse* **Dec**: 130–2

Byrne M (2002) Spirituality in palliative care: what language do we need? *Int J Palliat Nurs* **8**(2): 67–74

Calman K, Hine D (1995) A policy framework for commissioning cancer services. Report by the expert advisory group on cancer to the Chief Medical Officers of England and Wales. London: DoH

Carroll B (2001) A phenomenological exploration of the nature of spirituality and spiritual care. *Mortality* **6**(1): 81–98

Cawley N (1997) Towards defining spirituality: an exploration of the concept of spirituality. *Int J Palliat Nurs* **3**(1): 31–6

Cobb M (2001) *The Dying Soul.* Buckingham: Open University Press

DoH (2000) *The NHS Cancer Plan.* London: DoH

Draper P, McSherry W (2002) A critical view of spirituality and spiritual assessment *J Adv Nurs* **39**(1): 1–2

Dudley JR, Smith C, Millison MB (1995) Unfinished business: assessing the spiritual needs of hospice clients. *Am J Hosp Palliat Care* **12**: 30–7

Elsdon R (1995) Spiritual pain in dying people: the nurse's role. *Prof Nurse* **10**(10): 641–3

Govier I (2000) Spiritual care in nursing: a systematic approach. *Nurs Stand* **14**(17): 32–6

Hawkett A (1997) Directions in spirituality: a introduction to the theme. *Int J Palliat Nurs* **3**(1): 5

Hunt J, Cobb M, Keeley VL, Ahmedzai SH (2003) The quality of spiritual care-developing a standard. *Int J Palliat Nurs* **9**(5): 208–16

McEwen M, Wills EM (2002) *Theoretical Basis for Nursing.* Philadelphia: Lippincott Williams & Wilkins

McSherry W, Draper P (1996) The spiritual dimension: why the absence within nursing curricula? *Nurse Educ Today* **17**(5): 413–17

McSherry W (2000a) *Making Sense of Spirituality in Nursing Practice: an Interactive Approach.* Edinburgh: Harcourt Brace

Mc Sherry W (2000b) Education issues surrounding the teaching of spirituality. *Nurs Stand* **14**(42): 40–3

McSherry W, Ross L (2002) Dilemmas of spiritual assessment: considerations for nursing practice. *J Adv Nurs* **38**(5): 479–88

McSherry W, Cash K (2004) The language of spirituality: an emerging taxonomy. *Int J Nurs Stud* **41**(2): 151–61

Mayer J (1992) Wholly responsible for a part, or partly responsible for a whole? The concept of spiritual care in nursing. *Second Opin* **27**: 26–55

Markham I (1998) Spirituality and the world faiths. In: Cobb M, Robshaw V (eds) *The Spiritual Challenge of Health Care*. Edinburgh: Churchill Livingstone

Marstolf DS, Mickley JR (1998) The concept of spirituality in nursing theories: differing world-views and extent of focus. *J Adv Nurs* **27**: 294–303

Moss B (2002) Palliative care in acute hospitals. *Nurs Times* **98**(6): 35–6

Muncy JF (1996) Muncy comprehensive spiritual assessment. *Am J Hosp Palliat Care* **13**(5): 44–5

Murray RB, Zentner JB (1989) *Nursing Concepts for Health Promotion*. London: Prentice Hall

Naraynasamy A (1993) Nurses' awareness and preparedness in meeting their patients' spiritual needs. *Nurse Educ Today* **13**: 196–201

Naraynasamy A (1999) ASSET: a model for actioning spirituality and spiritual care education and training in nursing. *Nurse Educ Today* **19**: 274–85

Naraynasamy A (2001) Spiritual Care: a Practical Guide for Nurses and Healthcare Practitioners. 2nd edition. Wiltshire: Quay Books

National Council for Hospice and Specialist Palliative Care Services (1997) *Feeling Better: Psychosocial Care in Specialist Palliative Care*. London: National Council for Hospice and Specialist Palliative Care Services

National Institute for Clinical Excellence (NICE) (2004) Improving Supportive and Palliative Care for Adults with Cancer. London: NICE

Nolan P, Crawford P (1997) Towards a rhetoric of spirituality in mental health care. *J Adv Nurs* **26**: 289–94

Oldnall D (1996) A critical analysis of nursing: meeting the spiritual needs of patients *J Adv Nurs* **23**: 138–44

Pattison S (2001) Dumbing down the spirit. In: Orchard H (ed) *Spirituality in Health Care Contexts*. London: Jessica Kingsley

Piles C (1990) Providing spiritual care. *Nurse Educ* **15**(1): 36–41

Puchalski C, Romer AL (2002) Taking a spiritual history allows clinicians to understand patients more fully. *J Palliat Med* **3**(1): 129–37

Ross LA (1996) Teaching spiritual care to nurses. *Nurse Educ Today* **16**: 38–43

Rumbold B (2002) *Spirituality and Palliative Care*. Australia: OUP

Stoll R (1979) Guidelines for spiritual assessment. *Am J Nurs* **1**(9): 1572–7

Swinton J, Narayanasamy A (2002) Response to: Draper P, McSherry (2002) A critical view of spirituality and spiritual assessment [*J Adv Nurs* **39**: 1–2]. In: *J Adv Nurs* **40**(2): 158–60

Tanyi RA (2002) Towards clarification of the meaning of spirituality. *J Adv Nurs* **39**(5): 500–09

Taylor E, Highfield JM, Amenta M (1994) Attitudes and beliefs regarding spiritual care. *Cancer Nurs* **17**(6): 479–87

Taylor EJ (2003) Nurses caring for the spirit: patients with cancer and family caregiver expectations. *Oncol Nurs Forum* **30**(4): 585–90

Turner P (1996) Caring more, doing less. *Nurs Times* **92**(34): 59–61

Walter T (2002) Spirituality in palliative care: opportunity or burden? *Palliat Med* **16**(2): 133–9

WHO (1990) *Technical Report Series 804*. Geneva: WHO

Wright MC (2002) The essence of spiritual care: a phenomenological enquiry. *Palliat Med* **16**(2): 125–32

9

Sexuality and palliative care: a journey of discovery and understanding

Liz Searle

Part I

Introduction

If we accept that in palliative care, death is acknowledged, accepted and celebrated, that the approach to palliative care is holistic and includes psychosocial, physical and spiritual dimensions, then there is arguably nothing hidden. Care is delivered in settings by staff who pride themselves on including the whole family; on being non-judgmental; and on focusing on achieving a good death. What could possibly be missing?

The evidence, however, is damning. There is little literature on the topic of addressing sexuality with the dying; any existing literature concerns itself with the effects of different types of cancer and their biological impact. Some go as far as discussing fertility and survivorship issues, but there is virtually nothing written on the broader concept of sexuality (ie. broader than the act of sex) and even less on helping strategies for this particular group. The dying are being neglected in the provision of this area of care (Searle, 2002). In addition, personal experience of teaching groups of students studying palliative care reveals that little or no thought has been given to addressing this area of practice. This is not said critically. This would have been true of me when I was new to palliative care. In fact, it would have been true of general nursing practice. One could claim age and era as an excuse, but the same is true today.

It emerges that the reticence to discuss sexuality with the dying is not confined to the domain of nursing. Social workers equally find this a challenge (Neiman, 2002) and recently doctors have also been open about this complex issue (Yamey, 2001). In Neiman's study (2002), it is clearly thought to be the job of the multi-professional team — but who? Mixed successes in multi-professional working and communication leave sexuality buried under the more pressing work of team dynamics.

It's an indictment of the professions to discover that patient groups and in fact patients themselves are further up the learning curve. This is clearly evidenced by the internet (see 'Websites' section).

Finally, there are a few academic papers produced by practitioners, along with the articles on the biological effects of cancer. There is a claim of how well they address this issue of sexuality. However, with statements like, 'you have to ask the patient because they don't volunteer information', and without presenting a holistic definition of either sexuality or a counselling framework, healthcare professionals are left guessing as to the success of this intervention. But we are all learning and, if we let them, patients will share their expertise with us.

In conclusion, if dying is a part of life and sexuality a part of adulthood, and experience constitutes quality of life, 'hidden' sexuality can no longer remain.

Why is sexuality hidden?

I have made an assumption that sexuality is hidden, but there is also strong evidence to suggest this. But who is hiding what? Are patients hiding their needs from us, perhaps fearful of being judged. Or are we hiding our inability to cope with their sexuality, or to be helpful? The simple answer would be both, but, as this chapter will explore, it is much more complex.

'Hidden' happens when we don't understand, but mostly when we don't know, how to help. It is best not to travel that road with patients without a map, the directions, or the driving skills. Exploring the relationship between sex and death sounds like the world of dark backrooms and under-the-counter materials. Good palliative care is an art, more than a science. But bold and brave we must be if we are to make this issue in palliative care accessible and free to all. Some will appreciate the message, some will not; but increasing numbers will visit and stay longer, will try to understand what they see. Sexuality as part of palliative care is the contemporary era of health care.

This chapter will attempt to address the complex and often forgotten area of meeting the sexuality needs of dying patients. We will consider what it means to explore sexuality with this group of patients. What are the constraints, restrictions and boundaries? We will move on to consider a model of loss and its implications and applications to this issue. Searching for a broader and useful definition of sexuality, we will consider an adapted theory of love (Sternberg, 1986). This chapter is not the result of an evidence-based, empirical approach. The evidence is not yet there. It comes out of personal experience, anecdotal experience of esteemed colleagues, and patients and their families. I present this work as nothing more than a provocation — a contemplation and exploration of the possible issues that are yet to surface. I hope it motivates practitioners to begin to research this area further in search of evidence, and consider it broader than just the ability, or not, to have sex.

Although it is also important to consider aspects of symptom control, effects of frequently used drugs and the physical restraints on sexuality at this time of life, more attention will be paid to this issue in Part II of this chapter. Included at the end for further reading are some useful guides.

This chapter would not be complete without considering the culture and context within which much of palliative care takes place. The influence of this environment is perhaps the single most significant issue that effects the provision of holistic care. Without addressing this, or at least being mindful of it, little progress will be made.

This chapter aims not to give all the answers, but to raise awareness around sexuality and provoke thinking about our own practice and where this practice takes place — to consider the effects of attitude and the constraints of knowledge, but most importantly to promote a realisation that there is still much to do in this area of care.

Hidden behind a medical paradigm

In recent times, there has been a growing number of publications regarding the increased medicalisation of the dying (James and Field, 1992; Biswas, 1993). It is suggested that what was always considered good nursing care has grown in expertise and knowledge to palliative care and, more recently, specialist palliative care. This field is now well recognised as a specialty in nursing and medicine in its own right. Many would argue that this is rightly so and can only benefit the patient by concentrating skills, knowledge and research.

However, there remains a danger that a paradigm shift could occur away from viewing death holistically as a psychosocial experience to a more medical or biological focus. The skillful assessment and treatment of complicated symptoms may detract from more holistic care and open discussion of death and dying, which facilitates open communication and thus allows issues of sexuality to be explored.

Whilst the drive towards supporting cancer patients has continued, other diseases are gaining a higher profile: HIV and AIDS and to a lesser degree motor neurone disease and multiple sclerosis. It is increasingly more likely that people with these conditions may get access to palliative care services.

The number and range of services for people with coronary heart and vascular disease who may be facing death is less obvious, which is interesting when we consider that they remain the largest cause of death in the UK.

The long-awaited supportive care guidance from NICE is now with us. These guidelines are to ensure a standard of care is achieved. Sadly, early signs show little attention to sexuality.

So does the search for a cure and the medicalisation of diseases move us away from holistic care, thus undermining and delaying the journey towards exploring sexuality needs with patients? The current policy and political pressure on the healthcare system is a long list of 'must do's, measured by external agencies and scored as 'successes' or 'failures'. These 'must do's are as always numerically measured (bed occupancy, waiting times, and so on), whilst quality of care or communication is not given its rightful place. We are a long way from measuring how well holistic needs, including sexuality, are being met.

Sexuality and chronic ill-health

When we consider sexuality and in particular the act of sexual intercourse we often only imagine what is pertinent to our own experience. Sexuality is a social construct, influenced by culture, religion, familial and personal beliefs (Neiman, 2002). This experience is based on who we are, and on the powerful, often subliminal, messages we were exposed to. For example, if we are asked to imagine a pair of lovers, the picture we imagine may be of a young fit virile man and a slim young attractive female touching, kissing and cuddling. We are unlikely to picture a same-sex couple sitting on a park bench kissing, or an elderly couple watching a pornographic video, or a disabled woman manipulating her contorted body into a position that makes sexual intercourse possible, giving clear instructions to her new partner. Why? Because for many of us, it falls outside our own experience. It is not an automatic consideration and maybe difficult to imagine, even when provoked.

Yet for many, this is the real and challenging world; a personal world that may necessitate frequent contact with healthcare professionals in healthcare settings; a personal world where, just for once, it would be nice to be asked if their intimacy or sexual needs are being met.

Hidden or overexposed?

Part of our social construct is the influence of the media. Overexposure of unpleasant experiences such as death, violence and sexual deviance may lead to a numbing effect on us as individuals, or even create an unnatural interest. We may subliminally become less in touch with such tragedy or even fear reprisal if openly exploring such topics.

A recent book explored the issue of sex and death in the media (Pickering *et al* in Field *et al*, 1997). An interesting account of tabloid media coverage over a three-month period is presented. It shows us that death is frequently reported, but predominantly sudden, untimely death. The increased frequency of sexually related death and the presentation of those women who have died as young, sometimes even younger than they really were, portrays a skewed image of death. For example, the story of Marlene Dietrich, although she died in her nineties, was accompanied by a picture of her in her youth and at her height as a sex symbol. In addition, more attention was given to the deaths of young women where a sexual motive was suspected, or mutilation occurred. The time and space dedicated to these stories outweighed their frequency. The subsequent reporting of the reactions of the dead womens' male partners suggested a move from the traditional male stoicism to one of emotional wreck and turmoil.

The authors ask what can be gleaned from these data. Perhaps women should stay at home where their virtue can be protected? Perhaps these sexually motivated attacks on women raise female sexuality to a powerful, uncontrollable status, leaving men's masculinity threatened? Or perhaps death and sex are part of an unreal, over-produced play that encourages a sense of fantasy and voyeurism. Could the frequency of reporting and this media sensationalism put sex and death off the personally acceptable agenda for discussion and into the public domain only suitable to be discussed when it relates to others?

The tabloids are not the only places where references to death and sex are found. Over centuries, death and sex have been revealed in renowned works by authors such as William Shakespeare (1564–1616) and John Donne (1573–1631). In their works, death usually comes in the form of suicide. In Elizabethan times, both sex and suicide were forms of social and religious taboo. But the passion of forbidden love and sex found in, say, *Romeo and Juliet* may lead us to conclude that life without passionate love is so desolate that death can be the only release. So what can death be as the final stage of living if not to contain passionate love until the end? Scholars of John Donne argue that sex and death as concepts are used in his work interchangeably: both are extremes of excitement and fear.

Why then, we might ask, if sex and death have been part of our social environment for so long, can it be so difficult to address these important facets of life with the dying?

Generally, those who are dying, even where there are no obvious signs, are sexually disenfranchised (Siemens and Brandzel, 1982). Cancer is particularly desexualising (Sontag, 1979). For sick people, there are a number of expected ways to behave, a number of predicted needs identified among others by nursing models. The boundaries between patients and their professional carers are clearly defined. This could be summarised in the work describing the 'sick role' (Gorden, 1966). Being sick excuses the person from normal sexual activity. In acute illness, both the patient and the healthcare professional freely accept this asexual state. Historically, the preparation of nurses has focused on ill-health needs and getting patients home quickly, where they can resume their normal lives. A comfort zone therefore existed for both patient and carer where sexuality need not be addressed.

Yet when we explore the idea that not everyone will return to their previous health status, and indeed some may die whilst still retaining a need to live as complete and normal a life as possible, a new challenge emerges. Patients have a right to receive help, support and a non-judgmental attitude; to have their sexual needs acknowledged; and to redefine the boundaries between themselves and their professional carers. In return, it challenges healthcare professionals to search out knowledge and skills to meet these needs; to begin to offer holistic care to the chronically sick, disabled and dying by supporting their sexual needs; to do the unthinkable — to discuss sex with the dying.

Broadening our horizon — seeking understanding

The literature on terminally ill patients and sexuality is very limited. It often only explores reasons for the problems and focuses on the act of intercourse. However, although old, it is interesting to look at the work of Wasow (1977). During this study, terminally ill patients had a great need to talk about their sexual needs. Patients showed a strong need to continue their sexual relations. The benefit of sexual satisfaction and intimacy outweighed the pain, discomfort and drain on their energy. It is interesting that these findings have not been developed or further tested. However, the effects of the disease process cannot be underestimated. Apart from distressing symptoms, there are the effects of altered body image, disfiguring surgery and wounds, and the feelings the partner may have about not aggravating the disease or even catching it in the case of AIDS or, more mistakenly, cancer.

Sexual needs are clearly an important issue for people at the end of life. They have a need to feel loved; to belong; to share the most intimate of experiences with the one most important to them; to leave this world feeling that they may be missed, but more importantly that they made an impression.

Cancer is predominantly a disease of the older person. However, when cancer affects young heterosexual men, issues of sexuality suddenly play a leading role. The only examples of actively addressing sexual needs are found in the literature focused on this group: for instance, young men being found sympathetic prostitutes to enable then to experience sexual intercourse before they die is told without a blush in sight. Sperm banks, offered to those with high risk of becoming terminally ill to enable donation of life after death, have been given due attention (Grinyer and Thomas, 2001). How interesting that only here in this quiet backwater, suddenly, an openness and boldness can be found. Perhaps it is not so surprising if society considers young virile men as the pulse of its existence.

Defining unmet needs in people who are dying is clearly not straightforward. It depends on open and honest communication between the practitioner and the patient, and the patient and their partner. It is also dependent on the acknowledgment that the patient indeed has a partner in the case of same-sex couples or heterosexual couples engaging in extra-marital relationships. Most importantly, it depends on the idea that the lack of a partner does not equate to a lack of sexuality.

It is difficult to acknowledge that some people's lives are more complex than our own. Initiating a conversation around the topic of sexuality with a dying man who has met all his sexual needs for many years outside his marriage would certainly be enlightening. It may raise moral and ethical issues for practice if we consider facilitating this need. In addition, there may be feelings of guilt for a woman whose partner is now dying when she has been participating in extra-marital relationships. The continued fear of exposure for same-sex couples prevents an openness that would enable support to be offered. The Gay and Lesbian Medical Association urge for the training of healthcare professionals in being culturally competent in sexual minority status (see 'Websites' section). Furthermore, this association summerised recent research that indicated that lesbian, gay, bisexual and transgender people may be disproportionally affected by certain forms of cancer. Further study in this area will raise the expectation of these groups to health care delivered by practitioners who are knowledgeable and able to understand and offer support. Same-sex couples have tremendous difficulty in having their partner acknowledged and included in significant discussion of any kind. It is a brave and open couple who are able to state their next of kin as the same gender and also state their relationship as partner. For many, their secret lives continue.

Much of palliative-care provision has been funded and developed by organisations with strong Christian origins. Christian values may have lead to a controlling environment, which historically leads to sexuality being suppressed along with acknowledgement of same-sex relationships. This was evident when first the AIDS epidemic occurred. Many hospices refused at that time to take AIDS patients, even when they had Karposi sarcoma, reduced funding being the espoused fear. Same-sex couples were also refused the sacrament by the Church and felt obliged to hide their relationships at ceremonies such as funerals (Cave, 1993; Davenport-Hines, 1990; Giffen,1981). It is for these reasons that it is so important to push for the legal recognition of same-sex relationships.

In this chapter, the use of the word partner relates to homosexual and heterosexual couples.

More than just sex: an alternative model revealed — intimacy, passion and commitment

In addition to sexual difficulties are the psychological and emotional states of a dying person experiencing loss. To help us understand some of these problems, I am going to map Sternberg's theory of love (1986) with Stedeford's model of loss (1986). Whilst the strengths and weaknesses of both theories are important to reflect upon, they are used here merely as a framework to aid discussion.

Sexuality is defined in many ways. It is clearly not just the act of sexual intercourse or sexual expression. Perhaps a broader definition could be the giving and receiving of love. Working on this premise, Sternberg's theory of love has been adapted, redefining the central theme as sexuality. The theory is represented as a triangle (*Figure 9.1*).

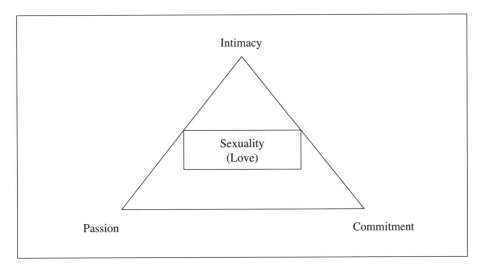

Figure 9.1: Sternberg's theory of love (adapted)

The suggestion here is that there are three main components to sexuality: passion, intimacy and commitment.

For the relationship to be satisfying, Sternberg would argue that there should be a close match between our own and our partner's triangle when placed together (*Figure 9.2*). However, each of the three components completing the triangle is defined uniquely by individuals. Therefore, what passion means to you and how you like it demonstrated is a matter for the individual. However, you have a need for your partner to match your own interpretation and therefore your needs; and, conversely, you theirs.

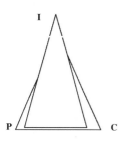

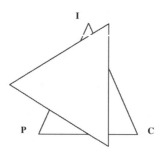

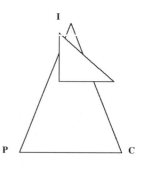

Well matched
(Same needs and ability to
demonstrate them)

Closely matched
(Some shared needs and ability
to demonstrate but need to
work together)

Mismatched
(Different needs
and abilities)

Figure 9.2: Interpretions of passion between partners

Each component must be defined and translated into action by both the individual and couple together. Complete understanding and action between couples leads to satisfaction. Difficulty in this process may lead to an unsatisfactory relationship. This may account for the often-used phrase, 'I know he\she loves me, I just wish he/she would show it'. To follow this to its ultimate conclusion, for healthcare professionals to help dying patients and their partners, they need to assess clearly what each component — intimacy, passion and commitment — means for each patient, and help them and their partner meet these needs or find alternate ways of doing so.

To complicate the picture further, we must consider the feeling of loss that both partners will be experiencing on the diagnosis and prognosis of an incurable disease which will lead to the ultimate separation. Stedeford's model (1986) has been selected on the basis of personal preference. Whilst it is inappropriate to elaborate on it here, I would recommend it as a work to consider. The basic framework is as follows: crisis of knowledge; shock numbness; psychological denial; anger (possible non-attention denial); and acceptance.

Mapping these two models allows us to explore specific difficulties in meeting sexual needs and suggest strategies for helpful interventions/advice.

Passion

The demonstration of passion from one partner to another may take many forms: touching, kissing, cuddling, requests for sexual activity, and intercourse itself. Through these actions, a clear message is given from one partner to the other. However, pre-occupation with other emotional work will inevitably reduce the ability to demonstrate or need passion. For example, on the diagnosis of an illness, the shock and numbness identified by Stedeford will clearly reduce the overall need for the full demonstration of passion, but may enhance the need for commitment and intimacy. Clearly, there may be a need to be reassured that the relationship is solid and will not falter. This timing may coincide with an admission to hospital where asexual status may be enforced.

It is vital that, on return home, as normal a relationship as possible is established. This can only occur if clear information is given to the couple regarding resuming sexual activity, the effects of certain medications, and practical advice on physical limitations. However, the shock and numbness felt by both partners are part of a process of anticipated loss (Worden, 1991), which is deemed essential in a normal grief reaction.

Stedeford suggests that a period of psychological denial may then occur along the lines of, 'It can't be happening' or 'It can't be me'. She argues that you can only deny something you are part way to believing. This denial, however, leads to a period of buffering when normality continues, while a slower acceptance can occur.

It would be reasonable to assume that where the demonstration of passion has resumed, it would continue here as if all is 'normal'. There will be a need to hold onto 'normality' for as long as possible, resuming where possible all activities. Failure at this time could lead to a heightened experience of loss, a compounded and enhanced realisation that all is not well. The increased stress will of course affect sexual expression, and may result in erectile difficulties for men and dryness or dyspareunia for women.

Passion — supporting strategies

Anxiety is often a self-fulfilling prophecy: 'fear of failure produces failure' (Hyda, 1994). The importance of support and understanding from the healthcare practitioner is vital. What is needed are clear explanations of the difficulties and encouragement to explore the areas in which demonstrating passion are possible. Understanding the effects of stress and advising on such matters as the use of lubricants might help ease the situation. Where symptom-control issues exist, then partner advice may help. Massage, for example, may be a demonstration of touch and tenderness and may also reduce the sensation of pain by creating a feeling of well-being, thereby blocking pain impulses.

The use of 'essential oils', particularly lavender or chamomile, to aid relaxation where acceptable may also compensate for odours that wounds and fungating tumours can produce. (However, as with any treatment, careful individual assessment should be carried out, including possible reactions to the oils.) Thus, touch can take place where it was once feared or unpleasant.

Clearly, for satisfying sexual activity to occur, the mind has to pay attention to the 'now' and not be preoccupied with the 'maybe'. Open discussion will often allow fears and anxieties to be explored.

The demonstration of passion can continue to its fullest up until the very last days of life. Feeling wanted and desirable may well be a relief from feelings of grief and depression. It is important to acknowledge and communicate to partners that one of the best therapies at this time is the one only they can give.

The demonstration of passion needs privacy and security. Patients spending large amounts of time in hospital or hospice settings have a right to this basic requirement. Many institutions are now considering internal locks on the doors of side-rooms with 'Do not disturb' signs. Many hospices have double beds in side-rooms. Yet there is much to do, particularly in the acute setting. It is as much about creating an environment of acceptance and non-judgmental attitudes as anything else. Healthcare professionals need to acknowledge the role of partners and recognise that patients are not asexual, but like all of us have sexual needs. Of course, no such attempts are being made to facilitate contact in acute settings: the culture here is much more focused on 'cure'.

Intimacy

The demonstration of intimacy takes the form of private and personal communications of feelings, personal information, emotional support and empathy. Giddens (1992) concludes that intimacy is therefore emotional communication.

One can clearly see where sharing intimacy with a partner may well facilitate the journey towards the acceptance of loss. The role for the healthcare professional may be in supporting the partner to support the patient.

Research on intimacy is limited. However, inventory tools such as Personal Assessment of Intimacy in Relationships (PAIR) (Schaefer and Olson, 1981) uses information such as:

- my partner listens to me
- my partner understands my hurts and joys.

Feelings of closeness and trust are important to this component of sexuality.

It is interesting to speculate on the effects on sexuality of the common scenario where the partner is told the diagnosis before the patient. Not only does this prevent the patient from beginning a normal and natural grief process, but it also immediately puts up barriers between the couple, which reduce the ability to demonstrate intimacy and hence, love. Fear of disclosing too much is a heavy burden for a partner to bear, particularly if their relationship is close. For those with less open relationships, it encourages collusion and withdrawal at a time when encouraging closeness would be preferable. I suspect little thought is paid to this undesirable situation and its impact on the patient's sexuality.

For the surviving partner, however, moving through a grief process in anticipation of the loss may also necessitate withdrawal of emotional support, a kind of damage limitation and a form of coping. Detachment of the partner too early in the dying trajectory leaves the patient with unmet needs. It is a challenge for the healthcare professional to support this emotional withdrawal while explaining this experience to the couple. The professional, through redefining boundaries, forms a trusting and therapeutic relationship and may be able to substitute the listening and emotional support needs of the patient, allowing a natural process of anticipated loss (Worden, 1991) for both.

Other stages identified by Stedeford, such as anger, will clearly impact on the demonstration of intimacy. We are often only angry with the people who truly understand us, in a safe environment. We think we can be angry because they will understand — but do they? Professionals explaining anger as a natural emotion and part of a grief process may help the patients' relationship to stay intact, facilitating understanding and allowing intimacy to continue.

Commitment

The third part of the triangle is commitment, described by Sternberg as 'seeing it through', 'accepting the good with the bad', the 'being with' someone, whatever the situation may bring.

As any healthcare professional will know, it is the 'being with' that often brings the greatest challenge. Watching a loved one die must be one of the most difficult experiences in life.

Clearly, no one could question the commitment of a partner who stayed throughout this situation, yet what choice do they have? Would society be accepting of someone who decided 'enough is enough'? When we think about it logically, in the cold light of day, of course we could not blame them for leaving. Yet comments such as 'they don't visit every day' or 'they hardly talk to each other' are said with negative connotations. Supporting partners to maintain and demonstrate their commitment is a vital role for the professional. Finding respite care when needed, or daycare, may bridge a divide before it widens.

As this section has developed, three main themes have evolved for consideration:

1. The importance of facilitating the needs of the patient in areas of intimacy and commitment; to support the partner's role, thereby facilitating sexuality needs.
2. To support the partner through communication and understanding to enable them to continue to demonstrate their love.
3. To acknowledge that patients without partners still have a need for intimacy and commitment.

Part II

Effects of sympton control and physical restriction on the sexual needs of dying patients — practical implications and tips

The combination of drugs often required to control symptoms will have a large impact on the meeting of sexual needs. Interestingly, in many symptom-control books, side-effects of drugs do not extend beyond morphine and constipation. Perhaps if you are dying, side-effects are considered irrelevant. The lack of information on this specific area leads us to speculate on possible effects of medication on sexuality. However, during that speculation, more work is clearly needed, but I would encourage healthcare professionals to observe and learn through their experience.

Pain relief

Many of the drugs used for pain relief result in constipation. The treatment of constipation is well-documented (Twycross, 1997; Regnard and Tempest, 1998). In addition, it is well-accepted to prescribe a laxative when prescribing these types of drugs, particularly opioids and weak opioids, such as codeine.

The effect of constipation on sexual function is obvious. It may make coitus for the woman uncomfortable, but for both genders the listlessness and nausea will result in lack of desire. For gay men, where anal intercourse is an important part of sex, constipation may be a vital problem to avoid.

Whilst it is recognised that the use of opiods for pain control in the terminally ill does not result in addiction, the only reference found to the effects of long-term use of opiates and sexuality is found in the literature studying abusers (Hollister, 1975). Opiates are found to severely depress sexual behaviour (Abel, 1985); in addition, erectile dysfunction may be common. Explanation of this possible side-effect is vital to couples, particularly if normal relations are to resume as soon as possible. There is a possibility that in the short-term, an increased sexual desire may occur as a result of freedom from pain and a feeling of well-being. This being the case, a window of opportunity exists for couples to affirm their relationship.

It would be interesting to consider the response of the healthcare team if a patient refused analgesia in favour of continued sexual function. This could only happen, of course, if the patient was able to make an informed choice. It would, however, represent the ultimate in patient empowerment.

Anti-cholinergic drugs used for drying secretions and occasionally nausea may cause erectile dysfunction, as they inhibit the parasympathetic nerves (Twycross, 1997). Sedatives used to induce sleep may also suppress desire and sexual response. However, tranquilisers and antidepressants may enhance sexual response by improving the patient's mental state. Clearly, the symptoms themselves may cause difficulties, and good symptom-control is paramount.

Patients in pain who feel nauseated and fatigued may not be able to fulfill or require a sexually active role. However, as described, love and the need for love are greater than sex. Expressing and receiving love is perhaps one of the greatest experiences. It is also never too late to learn. Even in relationships where love has not always been obvious, encouraging the demonstration of commitment may be helpful in facilitating grief for the remaining partner. Ambiguous and angry relationships are a risk factor for complicated grief reactions (Worden, 1991).

Physical considerations

Most of this chapter has discussed different approaches to sex and sexuality. However, there are some physical aspects to care that can be used to help the patient and loved ones live a near-normal life.

Syringe drivers

The use of syringe drivers for subcutaneous administration of medicines is now fairly common. The positions on which these are sited perhaps require a little more consideration. Couples who may wish to continue sexual activity or just wish to cuddle may find abdominal citing a problem. Upper chest, perhaps outer arm or leg, may be preferable although these too have their disadvantages.

Catheters

Catheters, whilst being cumbersome, affect the patient's feelings of sexuality and sexual freedom. For women, sexual intercourse may well be possible. Spigoting off the catheter is usually less restricting and minimises pulling and therefore trauma. Sexual intercourse is possible for catheterised men, again spigotted, although it may be uncomfortable. A condom placed over the top of the spigoted catheter prevents friction and therefore bladder trauma. Intermittent catheterisation may be possible leaving the catheter out for a short period, although this may of course be unacceptable to both.

Wounds

Fungating wounds are possibly one of the most difficult issues for patients and partners to address. It is a visual reminder of the disease process. However, it is important to remember that a partner may not see the same things we see. A partner sees and loves the whole person and their history, and may therefore be less shocked than anticipated. Charcoal dressings and, as mentioned, pleasant-smelling essential oils, are useful.

Breathlessness and physical impairment

Fear of increasing symptoms and even making the illness worse can restrict patients from experimenting with more comfortable positions. Finding positions that are not claustrophobic and include no undue increase in pressure and weight are those which are more upright, sitting or standing. Simple measures like emptying bowels and bladder, not eating a couple of hours before, and timing sexual activity to coincide with the peak of analgesic action, or just simply at the best time of day, can all make a difference. Many patients have other diseases that accompany old age, like arthritis and advice on these symptoms may also be necessary.

Becoming the carer — the hidden adult-to-adult relationship

It would be remiss not to address the altered dynamics within a relationship caused by the dependency of one partner and the need for the other to become the main carer.

A personal conversation with the wife of a man suffering from Alzheimer's disease epitomised this:

> *'I'm no longer his partner, sexual or otherwise. I'm his mother. I feed him, clean him, dress him, move him, toilet him. How can I then feel sexy towards him or meet my sexual needs? If I feel these needs are unmet, I feel guilty. He can't help it and I would never look elsewhere, if you know what I mean.'*

The field of transactional analysis (Berne, 1964) suggests we all fulfill adult-child and parent roles. These alternate with and perhaps complement our partners, resulting in the main or ideal with an adult-adult relationship. When either partner is sick, the other fulfills a parent role. When long-term serious illness forces a partner into a constant parent role, the likelihood of sexual activity resuming is reduced. 'One does not have sex with one's child' is a well-accepted social dictat.

Enabling partners to fulfill a more adult-to-adult relationship would perhaps facilitate sexual expression. Respite care is essential in this situation. If respite care or extra help can be arranged, it enables the partner to have time and space for themselves, thus enabling them to relinquish the parent role and prepare for a more adult sexual role. In the main, couples do not understand these dynamics, but a clearer understanding may be the route to a more fulfilling relationship.

Giving permission along with advice on creating the right environment is one of the most affirming things that healthcare professionals can do. Remembering that partners can support their loved one in life-affirming ways makes dying more a part of living. The following quotation, which is anonymous, makes this point with great eloquence:

> *In hospital, we sit together waiting for his death. Holding his hand does not help. We are alienated because I can no longer come to him with the love and nourishment of my body. We always used sex as a means of easing the tension of the day and giving us sustenance for tomorrow. Now all is lost. I feel that I have been denied my right to help him in a way no-one else can — in a way that no drug or doctor or nurse can help. Now I cannot ease his frustrations or give him proof of my love. I feel that I have abandoned him; that we are no longer facing his death together. I have failed him by letting his last days be away from home where there is no opportunity for physical closeness.*

Communication: hidden meaning

Can patients talk to us?

If openness is the key to successfully caring for the dying, then we must consider the obstacles that prevent this kind of relationship developing with our patients. The role of nurses as carers holds much in its history. The status of female nurses has swung between 'virgin' and 'whore'. However, the concept of 'angels' perhaps stems from images such as that of Florence Nightingale, 'The Lady with the Lamp', moving onto Victorian values of a good and proper job for a lady – a respected woman who took 'wifely obedience to the doctor and motherly concern to her patients' (Savage, 1987). One wonders how many nurses form parent-child relationships with their patients?

The further connotations of unmarried spinsters (presumably with little sexual experience) are of vocational, dedicated, asexual women. Add to this the sanctified status of nurses who care for the dying and a picture of purity is drawn. So how do patients talk openly about sexuality with these carers? Of course, this example is extreme to emphasise a point. But we must not underestimate the effects of environment, historical perceptions and stereotypes of nurses on the ability of patients to talk about intimate matters. 'Talking sex to angels' somehow challenges every preconceived notion that exists about professional relationships.

Clearly, developing a professional therapeutic relationship between professional and carer is not without its challenges. A reflective diary published by a therapeutic masseur elaborates on not crossing the boundary of therapeutic work into forming personal relationships (Van der Riet, 1998). Dress, language, posture and persona are part of reflecting on the use of 'self' as healer.

We know from earlier works that patients want to talk to us, want help and support, want to be freed from the fear of judgment. Perhaps we could view assessing sexuality needs as part of health education of the dying, along with symptom control and practical support? Sexual health could be viewed as a combination of somatic, intellectual, emotional and social aspects of sexual well-being (Penson, 2000).

Can we talk to patients?

We need to explore what can support good communications with our patients and be aware that there is an area of care that until now has been often forgotten. This care is broader than the act of sex and contains areas that can easily be supported and may make the most fundamental difference to dying well.

It is unlikely that patients need sex therapy. In a study by Tan *et al* (2002) of cancer patients referred for sexual counselling, 73% were seen only once or twice and needed basic advice and support. Sixteen percent were seen three to five times, and only a minority needed sex therapy, often stemming from problems long before their diagnosis.

Knowing what services are available in the local area for sexual counselling must be investigated, allaying practitioners' fears reported in the literature as an inability to help and a reticence to discuss the issue (Yaniv, 1995). Language is essential in talking to patients about such sensitive issues. Often the language used to describe sex sounds more like the Olympic Games than the domain of the dying (Yaniv, 1995). Personally, I find discussion around passion, intimacy and commitment an easier starting place.

We know little about the impact of a terminal illness on the sexuality needs of different cultural groups. Of the little work carried out, there are clearly differences. In an American study of women with early-stage breast cancer, Hispanic women showed significantly higher levels of concern around their sexuality needs compared with other women. The only conclusion that can be drawn is the importance of a unique, individual assessment (Spencer, 1999).

A useful guide to beginning to assess the needs of patients is the PLISSIT model (Annon, 1976):

> **P**ermission-giving
> **P**ermission to talk about concerns and needs
> **L**imited information
> **I**nformation: guides; sign-posting; basic information; clarifying causes
> **S**pecific suggestion
> **S**imple and complex advice and actions
> **I**ntensive therapy
> **T**herapy: domain of sex therapists

Conclusion

There is arguably so much to learn and understand about why sexuality remains a hidden dimension of palliative care. Palliative-care practitioners hold privileged places in the world of people who are dying. It is essential that we become bold and brave, and begin to explore this difficult yet essential area of care. Research must focus on how we can help and where differences can be made. There is also a role for education in making this topic acceptable to discuss in the classroom, and for reflective work to be valued and rewarded when it focuses on this issue.

This chapter has explored some of the issues that enable sexuality to remain hidden. I have tried to offer some supportive strategies to enable practitioners to be brave and begin to uncover this essential area of work. Sexuality can remain 'hidden' no longer. We all deserve better.

I would like to thank Blackwell Scientific who gave permission for the use of my earlier text from The Challenge of Sexuality in Health Care *(2002). In addition, I am grateful to the editors of that book, Hazel Heath and Isabel White, who were brave enough to let me publish and ordered my thoughts.*

References

Annon JS (1976) *Behavioral Treatment of Sexual Problems: Brief therapy.* Maryland: Harper & Row

Berne E (1964) *Games People Play.* London: Penguin

Biswas B (1993) In: Clarke D (ed) *The Future of Palliative Care: Issues of Policy and Practice.* Abingdon: Buckingham Press

Cave D (1993) In: Dickenson D, Johnson M (eds) *Death, Dying and Bereavement.* London: Sage

Davenport-Hines R (1990) *Sex, Death and Punishment.* Glasgow: William Collins & Sons

Giddens A (1992) *The Transformation of Intimacy.* Stamford: Stamford University Press

Gorden G (1996) *Role Theory and Illness.* New Haven: New Haven College and University Press

Griffin S (1981) *Pornography and Silence.* New York: Harper & Row

Grinyer A, Thomas C (2001) Young adults with cancer: the effect of illness on patients and families. *Int J Palliat Nurs* **7**(4): 162–4, 166–70

Hollister L (1975) The mystique of social drugs and sex. In: Sandler M, Gessa G (eds) *Sexual Behaviour: Pharmacology and Biochemistry.* New York: Raven

Hyda J (1994) *Understanding Human Sexuality.* USA: McGraw-Hill

James N, Field D (1992) The routinisation of hospice: charisma and bureaucratization. *Soc Sci Med* **34**(12): 1363–75

Neiman S (2002) *Sexuality, Cancer and Palliative Care: Research Perceptions and Practice of Social Work Staff in Central London Hospitals.* Monograph 192: Social Work Monographs. University of East Anglia: ISBN 1857840879

Penson *et al* (2000) Sexuality and cancer: conversation comfort zone. *Oncologist* **5**(4): 336–44

Pickering M, Littlewood J, Walter T (1997) In: Field D, Hockey J, Small N (eds) *Death, Gender and Ethnicity.* London: Routledge

Regnard CFB, Tempest S (1998) *A Guide to Symptom Relief in Advanced Disease.* Haigh & Hochland Ltd

Savage J (1987) *Nurse Gender and Sexuality.* London: Heinemann

Schafer M, Olson D (1981) Assessing Intimacy — the PAIR inventory. *J Marital Fam Ther* **8**(9): 47–60

Searle E (2002) Sexuality and the dying patient. In: Heath H, White I (eds) *The Challenge of Sexuality in Health Care.* Oxford: Blackwell Scientific

Siemens S, Brandzel R (1982) *Sexuality — Nursing Assessment and Intervention.* Philadelphia: JB Lippincott

Sontag S (1979) *Illness as Metaphor.* London: Penguin

Spencer SM (1999) Concerns about breast cancer and relationships to psychosocial well-being in a multiethnic sample of early stage patients. *Health Psychol* **18**(2): 159–68

Stedeford A (1994) *Facing Death, Patients, Families and Professionals.* 2nd edition. Oxford: Sobell Publications

Sternberg RJ (1986) Theory of love. *Psychol Rev* **93**: 119–35

Tan G *et al* (2002) Psychosocial issues, sexuality and cancer. *Sex Disabil* **20**(4): 22

Twycross (1997) *Symptom Management in Advanced Cancer.* Oxford: Radcliffe

Van der Reit (1998) The sexual embodiment of the cancer patient. *Nurs Inq* **5**: 248–57

Wasow M (1977) Human sexuality and terminal illness. *Health Soc Work* **2**(2): 105–21

Worden W (1991) *Grief Counseling — Grief Therapy.* New York: Springer

Yamey G (2001) Sexuality and cancer. *BMJ* **323**(i7317): 847

Yaniv H (1995) Sexuality of cancer patients: a palliative care approach. *Eur Int J Palliat Med Vol* **2**(2): 69–72

Websites

www.cancerbacup.org.uk

www.cancerbacup.org.uk/info/sex/sex-9.htm

www.mautnerproject.org — lesbians with cancer

www. glma.org/policy/hp2010/pdf/cancer.pdf — the gay and lesbian medical association

www.macmillan.org.uk — professional resources

Resources

Body Image — Sexuality and Cancer (1995) 4th edition. Cancerlink.
ISBN 1870534077

Close Relationships and Cancer (1998) Cancerlink. ISBN 01870534549

Sexuality and Cancer: for the Woman who has Cancer and her Partner (1988)
American Cancer Nursing Society

Sexuality and Cancer: a Guide for People with Cancer and their Partners (1995)
Cancerbacup. ISBN 1870403614

Sexuality and Cancer: for the Man who has Cancer and his Partner (1998) American
Cancer Society

10

The emotional load of caring: care for those for whom there is no cure

Heather Davies

Introduction

The idea of providing special care for those who are dying is not new. Institutions for the dying have been around since the late 1800s, providing care with the idea that no-one should die alone for the large number of people without family. Health care has improved, people live longer, families are smaller and more scattered, and the need for care for the dying to be given by those outside the family has increased. Although it is suggested that people would prefer to die at home, more people actually die in hospital and are not infrequently admitted shortly before dying (Hinton, 1994). Community health care and the availability of support for people to die at home is better than ever before, but perhaps within a few hours of death there is enormous stress for those who undertake the task of caring.

People who are dying have special physical, psychological, emotional and spiritual needs. Relatives and friends have significant challenges to face, which in turn impact on professional carers. Nurses are frequently in close daily contact with the patient and to understand the needs of the patient they must be able and willing to get involved at times at an emotional level. There is only one opportunity to do the right thing for someone who is dying and no opportunity to rectify mistakes for that individual after the event. Those who give palliative and terminal care also have personal needs, but because they are not dying, these needs are often overlooked. Whilst this may be manageable in the short term, prolonged exposure to grief and suffering can have a negative effect on carers unless steps are taken to ensure they are supported (Maslach, 1981; Maher, 1983; MacGuire, 1985).

Although the emphasis is now on openness and honesty about disease prognosis, death is not easily accepted in a world of advanced medical technology and treatment. Symptom control and the ability to keep very ill people alive is now so good that it is hard to determine when all palliation is exhausted and death is inevitable. High-technology care, cure or palliation of disease makes it difficult for people to accept that death is inevitable for everyone. The decision not to resuscitate can be difficult because symptoms may be reversible, although cure may not be possible. Death and expectations of how it should be managed have changed from being something discussed and accepted to something to be managed by other people and not talked about until absolutely necessary, and this may be within hours of the individual's demise. Maybe it is hard to care for someone who is dying within a hospital that is designed for curing disease, as death somehow suggests failure. This tends to be the case where there are two competing philosophies of care. There are simply not the resources in the fast pace of hospital health care to devote to patients who can often be helped only by time and painstaking attention to detail.

Caring for the dying involves families, friends and professional carers and will affect all these people in different ways. The rewards of looking after a loved one in the last stages of their life can be manifold. Children may feel they are repaying a debt to the parent who raised them. Staff involved in caring for the dying can gain enormous satisfaction from doing the job well. Conversely, someone who has recently been bereaved may have particular reasons for wanting to work with the dying, including previous experience of death not being handled well or family disease that has led to the death of family members, and may find looking after dying people difficult. This chapter will explore some of the issues for carers involved in palliative care.

Keeping mortality in perspective

There are a number of responses to working with the dying. There may be an over-identification, leading to sadness. There may be an avoidance of death by focusing on tasks and organisational rituals or the continuation of treatment, even when it is clear that no benefit can come of it. Dealing with people who are dying inevitably brings the idea of one's own mortality into perspective. It is no longer possible to think that death is something that happens to other people, and carers are faced with the stark reality that it could just as easily be themselves or their loved ones who are in the patient's place. In palliative care, there is more awareness of death. But whilst dying is part of life, it is not all that life is about. Coming to terms with death and keeping it in perspective are imperative if carers are to work with the dying without becoming overwhelmed.

Dealing with difficult emotions

The dying person and those who love them are arguably going through the grief process. Grief involves different emotions, including anger, guilt, depression, bargaining, denial and acceptance (Kubler-Ross, 1989). This range of emotions is not easy to deal with when only one person is experiencing them; complicate the mix to include families and friends and it can be very challenging. Patients can often deal with their emotions themselves or with their families if their well being is optimised by good clinical care. However, there are some emotions that have a direct impact on professional staff and are worthy of comment.

Denial or secrecy in the caring relationship can be hard to deal with, but may be necessary for the patient as part of the process of coming to terms with their own demise (MacGuire and Faulkner, 1988). Reality may be just too painful for the patient and it is not the right of the carer to force them to confront the truth if they are not ready or able to deal with it. If denial, optimism or not talking about negative things is the way the person has lived, they are not likely to change at the point of dying, and those who have known the patient prior to illness will have established communication patterns. However, denial is easiest for the patient and can be hard for everyone else involved. Staff may feel they are behaving dishonestly or colluding to keep reality from the patient. Friends and relatives may want to talk openly and say goodbye.

Anxiety and fear are not uncommon emotions experienced when an individual is close to death. Terror at the thought of imminent death can be hard for carers to watch, and if it is not well-managed with sedation, it can leave relatives and carers with memories that are difficult to endure. Many people do not reach a state of tranquil acceptance at their deaths. Fear and unrelieved symptoms can exacerbate their distress. It is important that all possible care is given quickly to palliate symptoms and psychological discomfort.

Anger is a normal emotion frequently experienced by the dying, their relatives and friends, and carers. Disbelief followed by anger is a common reaction when people are first given news of impending death, but anger can be experienced at any time. Anger may not always manifest openly but through manipulation, the over-demanding patient, or by depression if the anger is repressed. It is important to recognise that here anger may be the overt behaviour, but the hidden aspect is that there is blame being directed outwardly or externally at other people.

Healthcare staff often find anger difficult to deal with, even if they can understand that it is a normal and common response. Understanding that the patient has the right to be angry, staff may wonder how to deal with the strong feelings and be afraid that the anger may become uncontrolled (MacGuire, 1985). This can be especially so if the anger is aimed at members of the caring team who may be doing their best to provide good care and who they may feel the need to protect. It is important that the dying person is able to express their anger and other feelings, and that these are listened to and acknowledged. There are no 'right' answers or responses.

At the same time, carers have the right to say if the angry feelings become personal or a threat to their own integrity. However, deciding when to exercise this right, and how to do this knowing that the patient is ill and grieving, is difficult. Staff may feel that dealing with the patient's anger is a small price to pay for their own good health and guilty about their negative feelings towards the patient. Communication training is essential for professional carers who are likely to encounter these problems. Clinical supervision, mentorship and reflective practice can be helpful for clarifying feelings, gaining perspective and formulating coping strategies in this situation.

Closeness of the people involved

Professional staff, friends and family give care. The relationship and closeness of the people involved will affect their response. Health care staff will often have no knowledge of the patient prior to illness, and although they care and are involved, the person's death will not directly affect their personal lives. Relatives and friends are in a different position and their reactions and emotions are likely to be complex. In the case of prolonged illness, burn-out can be a problem and must be considered, and support given to reduce the risk. Burn-out describes a complex of psychological responses to the strain of constant interaction with people in need (Firth *et al*, 1996). Healthcare staff must deal with a variety of emotions from the patient and their friends and family, and if they have formed an attachment to the patient, they may have similar feelings.

The process of caring for the dying is inevitably intimate and may involve aspects of care not experienced even with their nearest and dearest. Partners who are involved with caring for each other or family members may undergo many different emotions related to care. The balance of their relationship is changed from interdependence to dependence. This will require adjusting to, as will undertaking intimate tasks previously performed by the individual.

Caring for someone who is dying can be time-consuming and, as death gets closer, often the one who is dying becomes less and less involved in the outside world and less able to have a truly reciprocal relationship with their loved ones. This can lead to feelings of loss and loneliness, even though the person is still alive. Death allows these feelings to be legitimately expressed. The person who is caring and not ill may feel guilty that they are well, especially if they indulge in unhealthy behaviour, or the patient is young or apparently blameless. They can be angry that their loved one has abandoned them by being ill and that they are no longer able to do the things they used to do. They often do not want to admit that they wish death would come soon, so that they can get on with their lives and move forwards.

While caring takes place, the rest of life slows down. Caring is a physically, socially and psychologically expensive activity, and the carer often has little time for other activities including looking after themselves. The death of the loved one can leave them with a large gap in their lives and socially isolated, having had little time to maintain their own social relationships. Additionally, if the caring has gone on for years as in the case of many degenerative diseases, grief may have been on hold and it may take some time before the bereaved is able to acknowledge their own pain and other negative feelings, start to grieve, and move on.

The death of someone to whom one felt close or cared for may result in a variety of emotions. There may be feelings of grief and loss, but also relief. Watching a loved one suffer is hard and it may be a relief when their misery is over. Relief that the person's suffering will end with their death is not unusual and is quite normal, but often causes guilt.

If the bereaved relied on the deceased for physical or emotional support or safety, there may be feelings of fear, excess anxiety and worry, as well as hopelessness and helplessness (Parkes and Weiss, 1983). Where there has been significant conflict in the relationship, especially in spousal relationships, there is less anxiety, depression, guilt and yearning for the deceased (Parkes and Weiss, 1983). Ambivalence in the feelings towards the deceased are also problematic. It can be more socially acceptable to admit to feelings of ambivalence towards a parent than towards a child or spouse, and this too affects how quickly the bereaved comes to terms with the death.

The difficult emotions that are raised when someone who is loved is dying can lead to greater emotional depth and development, but can also lead to fear of getting involved emotionally in case the pain felt at losing the person is experienced again. Arguably, to have no pain when dealing with the dying can mean that there is no-one the carer cares about. However, to care also means that death can be painful and burn-out a problem.

Aspects of care: what makes another person feel cared about?

The challenge of helping someone feel cared about is significant. Suffering is highly individual (Cassell, 1992; Van Hooft, 1998). Every person has different things that make them feel better, and these are often rooted in childhood or personality (Beck, 1988).The carer has a difficult job to do in determining what actions help a person feel cared for. Good symptom control may be the most helpful intervention, as it will help enable the person to process their feelings by themselves or with their loved ones. Caring for people at the end of their lives is complicated by the fact that there may be no opportunity in the future to rectify any mistakes.

Gaut (1983) identifies three necessary and sufficient conditions whereby an action could be described as caring:

1. Having knowledge about the patient to identify that care is needed and knowledge about what to do.
2. Implementing an action based on knowledge.
3. Evaluating the benefit of the action on the patient.

These conditions reinforce the view that nursing must have a holistic approach to patient care and that for caring to take place, the patient must be assessed and their care planned, implemented and evaluated based on their individual needs. In considering the meaning of suffering to individual patients, the person's response to their plight is crucial and carers must take this into account.

Nurses undertake many activities that are centred on caring for the patient, which range from providing physical help with the tasks of daily living to emotional support for the patient who is frightened or anxious about what is happening to them. Research into what helps people cope show four main components (Cutrona *et al*, 1986):

- emotional support
- information or advice
- material support
- instrumental support.

However, activities that nurses think help patients are not the same as those identified by patients themselves. Nurses often focus on the relationship between the nurse and patient as being important in helping the patient, whilst patients often state that what helps them are interventions that relieve specific problems (Smit and Spoelstra, 1991; Schukla and Turner, 1984; Widmark-Peterson *et al*, 2000). This wide difference in perceptions may mean that often the nurse is trying to help in a way that is not appreciated and may miss out on activities that are. This can lead to feelings of inadequacy in the nurse as their best efforts go unnoticed and not regarded.

The challenge of caring

Individualised care is dependent on assessing and identifying the patient's needs. Acceptance that things that help the patient may come from clinical knowledge and experience, and that these may be more important than focusing on the patient's psychological difficulties, may be realised only with experience and reflection.

Some caring staff are better than others at patient assessment and some patients will prove easier to assess. Experience and the personal attributes of the carer may colour their ability to assess the patient and thus identify what aspects of mind or body dysfunction are causing distress. The lessening of symptoms does not always result in relief of suffering, and what will help one patient will not help another. Therefore, tailoring care to meet the individual's needs is crucial, and individualising care means having more than a superficial knowledge of the patient and knowledge of symptom relief. Roach (1984) proposed that caring arises from a deep interest in humanity, a view echoed by Benner and Wrubel (1989) that 'caring is a basic way of being in the world'. Involvement and interaction with the patient are necessary for this type of caring to take place. The routines of task-orientated care miss the essential component of the relief of suffering as they are not individualised to the patient's needs.

There seems to be a difficult balance to be achieved between being involved with the patient whilst maintaining a level of clinical detachment that allows problems to be judged in a way that eliminates personal bias and is based on the patient's needs. Cassell (1992) discusses the loss of central purpose that arises when a person is suffering, and goes on to explain that to overcome suffering the person must be helped to reintegrate into their life. The thorough assessment of the patient, leading to the identification of what will help, requires commitment and involvement. Compassion and empathy are crucial in understanding the patient's viewpoint and what will help them respond to the threat to their integrity. What makes professional carers wish to be involved with the patient and how do they cope with continued exposure to suffering that cannot be relieved?

The empathic response

What motivates carers to spend time assessing the patient's needs, and establishing what problems are causing suffering, may be considered from both psychological and biological viewpoints. Psychologically, in order that human beings live harmoniously together, cooperation and helping behaviours are necessary. The motivation for these behaviours could be classed as empathy and the desire to do one's best towards others. This view assumes that human beings are able to understand what someone other than themselves may be feeling and respond to them in a positive way. A degree of empathy and compassion seems to be required to decide what would be a helpful response to an individual requiring assistance.

In a biological sense, there is evidence that the brain structures required for a primitive affective involvement with others were present in early human evolution (MacLean, 1958) and empathy could therefore have contributed to human social existence and the continuation of the species. The exposure of human beings to danger has been prevalent throughout history, and often individuals have a better chance of overcoming threat to their well-being if they unite to fight a common enemy. The tendency to help others in distress may be part of our biological inheritance.

Empathy is necessary to understand another human being, and seems to be essential to identify what suffering means to the person. Compassion motivates us to alleviate distress (Orlando, 1972; Carver and Hughes, 1990; Reynolds and Scott, 2000). In palliative care, empathy is crucial and it is possible that this is one of the reasons that caring for this group of patients is so difficult and exacts a considerable emotional toll.

Numerous studies have shown that there is a lack of empathy shown by the caring professions (MacLeod-Clarke, 1983; Hughes, 1990; MacKay *et al*, 1990). Lack of time, support, education and supervision have been given as reasons (Melia, 1981). Empathy requires a range of human emotions. Inexperienced carers may find it difficult to feel empathetic due to insufficient exposure to the different situations experienced by patients. Cues that people give to illustrate their distress affect the level of empathetic response from the carer and a different account of experienced problems may be given to those with whom they have no emotional involvement. People often want to protect those they know will be distressed by their discomfort and so do not always give a full description of problems.

The carer may respond to situational cues as well as to patient cues. Knowledge of disease processes will allow anticipation of suffering in the patient before the patient becomes aware of it. Although this may allow the carer to respond to prevent or alleviate suffering, arguably it is not individualised care based on the patient's needs, as care is then determined based on knowledge rather than on the patient's account. The carer needs to separate his or her own response to a situation from the patient's response, so that care is tailored to the patient's feelings. There are difficulties in achieving truly person-centred care, and a need for sharing care and not becoming so emotionally involved that objective and individualised patient assessment becomes coloured by prior knowledge or personal feelings.

Nurse involvement

The nurse-patient relationship has been hailed as the cornerstone of professional nursing practice (Pearson, 1988; Salvage, 1990; Morse, 1991; Wright, 1994; Savage, 1995). There are advantages to professional involvement in that it can provide job satisfaction and personal fulfilment whilst providing the patient with someone to confide in, gain support from, and trust during a stressful time. There are also disadvantages, including the patient relying too heavily on the carer and emotional pain for the carer (Turner, 1999). Morse (1991) highlights the dangers of becoming over-involved whilst Wright (1994) believes that nurses should set clear limits to their involvement. Menzies (1961) identified that very strong mixed feelings are aroused in the nurse: pity, compassion and love; guilt and anxiety; hatred and resentment of the patients who arouse these strong feelings; and envy of the care given to the patient. She maintained that 'nursing patients with incurable diseases is one of the nurse's most distressing tasks'. Davitz and Davitz (1975), exploring how nurses felt about patients suffering, reported feelings of helplessness, inadequacy, depression, despair and anger. However, Field (1984), also exploring nurses' feelings about dealing with dying patients, found that whilst caring for this group of people is not always easy, it is also rewarding as it allows nurses to implement fully their ideal of nursing care.

Inevitably, there are some patients with whom the carer will have a greater bond or understanding, and the involvement may lead to pain and loss when the patient dies. Conversely, there are some patients who are disliked or whom the carer tends to avoid. Accepting that it is not possible to like everyone, and that good care can be given even to those who are disliked, is important. A balance that allows one to care without becoming over-involved requires self-knowledge and the ability to say 'no'. The unpredictability of relationships between nurses and patients makes the nature of their involvement difficult to teach. However, theory has a predictive role and can demonstrate what happens if nurses become over-involved with patients.

There is little literature on how nurses are to manage their personal involvement. In her research into the nurse-patient relationship, Turner (1999) found that less experienced nurses were less able to control their level of involvement with patients, whilst those with more experience employed two particular strategies:

1. **Setting boundaries**: this enables nurses to make a conscious decision about how far they will take their personal involvement.

2. **'Switching off'**: the nurse stops thinking about work when she goes home and is able to get on with her life outside work.

Turner (1999) developed a 'theory of managing involvement' and suggests that involvement needs to be kept within the boundaries of a professional relationship if it is to be sustainable. The more experience nurses have, the better they are at managing their involvement and this seems to be based on their level of experience and knowledge. As they develop maturity, they become more aware of the effects of their behaviour, both on themselves and on those around them (Turner, 1999).

Altruism and the effect of non-response to care

What happens if the patient fails to respond to the care being given and continues to suffer? The carer may also be satisfying personal needs in helping the patient, and this may affect how much effort is put into assessment and care. There is evidence that altruistic action may require a certain amount of need-fulfilment in the helper. This is so they can become more aware of the person they are helping and less aware of their own response to the situation — and thus better able to respond to cues being given out by the person they are trying to help (Hoffman, 1977). Concerns about failure, physical discomfort, or lack of knowledge about how to help may adversely affect the carer's ability to care. These factors will be enhanced if the person fails to respond to actions aimed at relieving their suffering. Continued suffering on the part of the person in the face of helper intervention has been shown to have an adverse effect on the carer's continued positive response to their plight and the desire to continue to help the individual (Hoffman, 1977; Lorber, 1974; Kelly and May, 1982). Nurses will often return to task-orientated non-involved caring of the patient if the patient fails to respond positively to interventions. This seems to be a form of self-protection on the part of the nurse against burn-out or personal suffering when the care being given is not helpful or the patient is dying (Forrest, 1989).

Caring activities that centre around addressing biological needs continue until death, and ensuring that these needs are met will reduce patient suffering. Unrelieved suffering may be due to intractable symptoms or because the person is dying. It is therefore important to mitigate carer stress if they are exposed to continual suffering. The carer must find a way to cope with this if he or she is to continue to give the same attention to every patient that the relief of suffering seems to require (MacGuire, 1985; Turner, 1999).

The harm that caring can do

Death and dying is one of the most stressful areas of care (Menzies, 1970; Turner, 2001; Davitz and Davitz, 1975). There is no right way to die and not all situations can be tidily resolved. Some people will die still not accepting the inevitability of death or having come to terms with their lives. Awareness is crucial to avoid the situation whereby the carer is trying to compensate for situations where things did not work out as they would have liked. Reparation for previous events, where the carer tries to ensure that the dying person has a 'good death', can lead to attempts to coerce the dying person to reach a point of acceptance about their own demise that they may not really feel. Carers can often feel overwhelmed by the complexity of care, both psychological and physical. If unable to alleviate distressing symptoms due to inadequate knowledge, the carer may also feel inadequate and helpless.

The 'helping profession syndrome' (Malan, 1979), where carers devote their lives to giving care and concern to others that they want for themselves, or 'compulsive care-giving' (Bowlby, 1980), may motivate carers to take on more and more caring work and to be overprotective of patients, disregarding their personal time limits or self-caring and resulting in burn-out. Maher (1983) describes a composite syndrome including exhaustion, psychosomatic illness, insomnia, negative attitude to clients and work, use of alcohol or other drugs, altered self-concept, guilt, pessimism, apathy and depression. Maslach *et al* (1981, 1982) focuses on three processes centred on loss of respect for patients. These are emotional exhaustion, depersonalisation and perceived lack of personal accomplishment. Cherniss (1980) clarifies the difference between burn-out and temporary fatigue or strain. All definitions have in common the feelings of ineffectiveness and futility, giving up all attempts to improve things and increasing conformity and rigidity. Besides the harmful effects on the carer, this type of behaviour can lead to other staff and the patient's family and friends feeling inadequate and left out, which will have an isolating effect on both them and the patient.

Often there is a public expectation that palliative care staff are somehow different or special — a feeling sometimes perpetuated by the staff themselves. This can lead to reluctance to admit when caring is too much and a break is needed. There is conflicting evidence about nurse stress in palliative care. Some studies show no more stress than other areas of care (Vachon, 1987, 1995) and others that nurses are more stressed (Bene *et al*, 1991; Cooper *et al*, 1990).

The importance of hope

Medical services in general continue to regard death as something to be resisted, postponed or avoided (Clarke, 2002). Acute medicine is concerned with the patient's recovery and can often interpret death as a failure. Quality of life is the essence of palliative care philosophy. Relationships that are formed bring hope to scenarios that seem desperate and empty of any possibility (Hennezel, 1997). For those who specialise in caring for the dying, hope lies in accepting the inevitable and supporting the individual to acceptance or being realistic about the impending death.

A sense of helplessness in the professional is equated with a sense of hopelessness in the patient (Chaplin and McIntyre, 2001). To enable patients can restore a sense of hope for both the patient and the professional. However, for hope to be effective it has to be active and not passive (Hockley, 1993). Hope will lead to an action and the setting of goals — and action towards goals themselves (Carson, 1989). A person with active hope may be more willing to participate in achieving important, realistic and significant goals. Nursing is about helping people to achieve their needs when they are unable to do this for themselves (Henderson, 1966; Royal College of Nursing, 2003). If nurses are unable to help the patient, this can result in the nurse feeling inadequate and demonstrates that helplessness can lead to hopelessness.

Hope seems to be an important aspect of caring for people when they are terminally ill as it helps carers to transcend the present situation by having a sense of purpose and fostering a positive new awareness of being (Herth, 1990). In the professional, it is this awareness that can have an impact on practice and contribute to their coping mechanisms. Farran *et al* (1995) suggest that hope and coping are inextricably linked; Weisman (1979) argues that hope is a prerequisite for effective coping. Hope is identified as a strategy for coping; as an emotion-focused and problem-solving approach; and as a method of cognitive appraisal (Lazarus and Folkman, 1984). Problem-focused coping depends on modifying or changing the situation to bring about improvement. Emotion-focused coping is the ability of the individual to alter the perception of the situation and to reduce the amount of stress it causes. Employing hope as a means of appraisal provides a strategy for professionals, not only to enhance their care but also as a way of caring for themselves.

Support systems

A number of factors has been shown to help staff involved in intense caring work. There is an important role for educational strategies such as guided reflection, clinical supervision and mentorship in enabling nurses to learn about and manage their involvement.

Meutzel (1988) argues that nurses need to be supported in multiple ways and need professionally facilitated staff support as well as ad-hoc caring interactions between nurses. Johns (1990) advocates clinical supervision and Menzies (1961) and Benner and Wrubel (1989) argue that instead of avoiding anxiety, nurses need to learn how to confront it and to do this they need structured help and support.

Role models who can demonstrate involvement and caring whilst looking after themselves and recognising their limitations are a valuable resource for new or inexperienced carers. The management style of clinical leaders will determine whether they will become a positive or negative role model and the level of support provided (Smith, 1992).

Professional carers need to be equipped with the knowledge and skills to care for patients who have complex needs and to manage the patient relationship. Difficulties can arise from lack of knowledge and skills about how the patient can be helped. Education and training should therefore be aimed at how best to alleviate symptoms as well as understanding the emotional, spiritual and psychosocial issues in caring for the dying. Education should include how to recognise situations, anticipate them, react to them, and intervene effectively and take lessons for the future. Clinical supervision is important and should involve reflection with a supervisor who not only listens to the carer's feelings, but also helps to identify what knowledge and skills must be learnt to develop care for the future. All those involved in palliative care should undergo communication and coping-skills training. Often the best emotional support that can be given to those involved in caring for the dying is ensuring that their knowledge and skills enable them to alleviate distressing symptoms and understand the patient's grief and any psychological distress.

Palliative care can be rewarding and can enable carers to mature and grow. However, it is complex and burn-out is a significant hazard. Understanding and good support systems are imperative to avoid the negative aspects of care.

References

Beck AT (1988) *Love is Never Enough.* New York: Harper Row

Benner P, Wrubel J (1989) *The Primacy of Caring, Stress and Coping in Health and Illness.* CA: Addison-Wesley, Menlo Park

Benner P (1994) *Interpretative Phenomenology. Embodiment, Caring and Ethics in Health and Illness.* Thousand Oaks, London, New Dehli: Sage

Bene B, Foxall MJ (1991) Death anxiety and job stress in hospice and medical-surgical nurses. *Hosp J* 7: 25–41

Bowlby J (1980) *Attachment and Loss.* Vol. 3. New York: Basic Books

Carson VB (1989) Spiritual Dimensions of Nursing Practice. Philadelphia: Saunders Co.

Carver E, Hughes J (1990) The significance of empathy. In: MacKay R, Hughes J, Carver E (eds) *Empathy and the Helping Relationship.* New York: Springer Publishing Co.

Cassell EJ (1992) The nature of suffering: physical, psychological, social and spiritual aspects. In: Kinghorn S, Gamlin R (eds) *Palliative Nursing: Bringing Comfort and Hope.* London: Balliare Tindall

Clarke EJ (2002) Between hope and acceptance: the medicalisation of dying. *BMJ* **324**: 905–7

Cherniss C (1980) *Professional Burnout in Human Service Organisations.* New York: Praeger

Cooper CL, Mitchell S (1990) Nursing the critically ill and dying. *Human Relat* **43**: 297–311

Cutrona CE, Russell D, Rose J (1986) Social support and adaptation to stress by the elderly. *Psychol Aging* **1**: 47–54

Farran C, Herth K, Popovitch J (1995) *Hope and Hopelessness*. London: Sage

Field D (1984) 'We didn't want him to die on his own': nurses' accounts of nursing dying patients. *J Adv Nurs* **9**: 59–70

Firth H, McIntee J, McKeown P, Britton P (1986) Burnout and professional depression: related concepts? *J Adv Nurs* **11**: 633–41

Forrest D (1989) The experience of caring. *J Adv Nurs* **14**: 815–23

Gaut DA (1983) Development of a theoretically adequate description of caring. *West J Nurs Res* **5**(4): 313–34

Herth KA (1990) Fostering hope in terminally ill people. *J Adv Nurs* **15**: 1250–9

Henderson V (1966) *The Nature of Nursing*. New York: Macmillan Publishing Co.

Hennezel M (1997) *Intimate Death*. Warner Books

Hinton J (1994) Can home care maintain an acceptable quality of life for patients and their relatives? *Palliat Med* **8**: 183–196

Hoffman ML (1977) Empathy: its development and prosocial implications. *Nebr Symp Motiv* **25**: 169–217

Hughes J, Carver E, MacKay R (1990) Learning to have empathy. In: MacKay R, Hughes J, Carver E (eds) *Empathy and the Helping Relationship*. New York: Springer Publishing Co.

Johns C (1990) Autonomy of primary nurses: the need to both facilitate and limit autonomy in practice. *J Adv Nurs* **15**: 886–94

Kelly MP, May D (1982) Good and bad patients: a review of the literature and a theoretical critique. *J Adv Nurs* **7**: 147–56

Kinghorn S, Gamlin R (eds) *Palliative Nursing: Bringing Comfort and Hope*. London: Balliare Tindall

Kubler-Ross E (1989) *On Death and Dying*. London: Tavistock

Lazarus RS (1966) *Psychological Stress and the Coping Process*. New York: MacGraw-Hill

Lazarus RS, Folkman S (1984) *Stress, Appraisal and Coping*. New York: Springer Verlag

Lorber J (1974) Good patients and problem patients: conformity and deviance in a general hospital. *J Health Soc Behav* 213–25

Maher EL (1983) Burnout and commitment: a theoretical alternative. *Pers Guid J* **62**: 390–4

Malan D (1979) *Individual Psychotherapy and the Science of Psychodynamics*. London: Butterworths

MacGuire P (1985) Barriers to psychological care of the dying. *BMJ* **29**: 1711–13

MacGuire P, Faulkner A (1988) Communication with cancer patients: 2 Handling uncertainty, collusion and denial. *BMJ* **297**: 972–4

MacKay R, Hughes J, Carver E (1990) *Empathy in the Caring Relationship*. New York: Springer Publishing Co.

MacLean PD (1958) The limbic system with respect to self-preservation and the preservation of the species. *J Nerv Ment Dis* **127**: 1–11

MacLeod-Clarke J (1983) Nurse-patient communications: an analysis of conversations from surgical wards. In: Wilson-Barnett J (ed) *Nursing Research: Ten Studies in Patient Care*. Winchester: Wiley

Maslach C, Jackson S (1981) The measurement of experienced burnout. *J Occup Behav* **2**: 99–113

Melia K (1981) Student nurses' construction of nursing: a discussion of a qualitative method. *Nursing* **77**: 697–9

Menzies EP (1970) *The Functioning of Social Systems as a Defence against Anxiety*. London: Tavistock

Muetzel PA (1988) Therapeutic nursing. In: Pearson A (ed) *Primary Nursing: Nursing in the Burford and Oxford Nursing Development Units*. London: Croom Helm Ltd

Morse JM (1991) Negotiating commitment and involvement in the nurse-patient relationship. *J Adv Nurs* **16**: 455–68

Orlando I (1972) *The Discipline and Teaching of the Nursing Process*. New York: Putman

Parkes CM, Weiss RS (1983) *Recovery from Bereavement*. New York: Basic Books

Roach MS (1984) The human mode of being: implications for nursing. In: *Prospects of Caring Monograph*. University of Toronto, Canada: Faculty of Nursing

Pearson A (1988) (ed) *Primary Nursing: Nursing in the Burford and Oxford Nursing Development Units*. London: Croom Helm

Reynolds WJ, Scott B (2000) Do nurses and other professional helpers normally display much empathy? *J Adv Nurs* **31**(1): 226–34

Salvage J (1990) The theory and practice of the 'New Nursing'. *Nurs Times* **86**(4): 42–5

Savage J (1995) *Nursing Intimacy: An Ethnographic Approach to Nurse-Patient Interaction*. Harrow, London: Scutair

Shulka RK, Turner WE (1984) Patients' perceptions of care under primary and team nursing. *Res Nurs Health* **2**: 93–9

Smit J, Spoelstra S (1991) Perceptions of caring: do patients and nurse agree? *Caring* **10**: 34–6

Smith P (1992) *The Emotional Labour of Nursing: its Impact on Interpersonal Relations, Management and the Educational Environment in Nursing*. London: Macmillan

Starck P, McGovern J (eds) *The Hidden Dimension of Illness: Human Suffering*. New York: National League for Nursing Press

Turner M (1999) Involvement or overinvolvment? Using grounded theory to explore the complexities of nurse-patient relationships. *Eur J Oncol Nurs* **3**(3): 153–60

Turner M (2001) Managing Involvement: a Grounded Theory of Nurse Personal Involvement in Relationships with Cancer Patients. Unpublished PhD

Vachon MLS (1987) *Occupational Stress in the Care of the Critically Ill, the Dying and the Bereaved*. New York: Hemisphere Press

Vachon MLS (1995) Staff stress in hospice/palliative care: a review. *Palliat Med* **9**: 91–122

Van Hooft (1998) Suffering and the goals of medicine. *Med Health Care Philos* **1**: 125–31

Weisman AD (1979) *Coping with Cancer*. New York: McGraw-Hill

Wright SG (1994) *My Patient-My Nurse: The Practice of Primary Nursing*. 2nd edition. London: Scutari Press

Widmark-Peterson V, Von Essen L, Sjoden PO (2000) Perceptions of caring amongst patients with cancer and their staff: differences and disagreements. *Cancer Nurs* **1**: 32–9

11

The final word

Brian Nyatanga, Maxine Astley-Pepper

Introduction

The preceding chapters clearly identify numerous aspects of palliative care that are hidden. Each of the contributors has focused on an aspect they believe remains hidden and in doing so have outlined some of the realities and intricacies of death and dying in palliative care. Through this frank discussion, it is hoped that healthcare professionals may begin to challenge openly their own perceptions and influence in the delivery of care.

In this summary, we aim to highlight areas that needed further discussion: the positive aspects of dying; death and the role of funeral directors in perpetuating these positives; the power of death; and the irony of death-denial.

We are aware that there are many other hidden aspects in palliative care, some of which are beyond the scope of this book. What we can do is remind the reader of certain aspects in order to begin to think of the best ways of managing and delivering sensitive palliative care. It has been argued that there may be a discrepancy in the care provision for those dying outside a specialist palliative-care setting. This group has been referred to as the 'disadvantaged dying' (George and Sykes, 1997).

It is still evident that black and minority ethnic groups do not always access palliative care services, and the reasons for this apparent reluctance remain ill-understood or even hidden. There are issues of language, cultural beliefs, values and perceptions of health that also need understanding by professionals providing these services. It is important that policy-makers and educators are particularly aware of the different cultural needs in order to provide services that respond effectively and sensitively to them.

The positive aspects of dying

This book has attempted to highlight hidden aspects and dispel some of the myths in caring for the dying. However, we are aware that there may be positive elements for the dying person that have not yet been acknowledged. Consideration of these elements may be uncomfortable for some, so we intend to draw them into sharper focus as sensitively as possible.

It may now seem natural for a dying person in the UK, or most western societies, to receive every care possible from the moment they are given a cancer diagnosis. Such care and resources would not be available if dying was not an inevitable part of this prognosis. The knowledge that someone is dying makes people around that person change their outlooks and relationships with him. There is a tendency for most healthcare professionals (in hospice and palliative-care settings in particular) to become 'unnecessarily nice' to the dying person (Street, 1995). There is no other plausible explanation for this, apart from the fact that the person is dying. It seems that when one is dying, all is forgotten and forgiven. The dying person is literally allowed to do as he pleases, and every attempt is made to grant his wishes.

The sudden adoption of a such a *laissez-passer* attitude may be to give the dying a smooth passage into death (Van Gennep, 1961). The work of Van Gennep considers three 'phases' in such a passage — separation, transition and incorporation — and only positive comments and attributes are thought to facilitate this movement through these phases. (For further detail of this process, see Nyatanga [2001].) Have you ever wondered why, at funeral ceremonies, only the good, positive aspects of the dead are highlighted, whilst any negative points are completely overlooked? Van Gennep (1961) argues that the intended outcome of this behaviour is that the dead can be incorporated and integrated into a new social order. However, such understanding may not be generally shared or acknowledged by relatives, friends and some professionals as the motive behind their behaviour towards the dying patient. If this was not the explanation, what rationale could be proffered as an alternative?

The knowledge that someone is dying often results in family members resolving their differences before the person dies, and one wonders why this is so important. Where relationships had been strained, dying could be seen as the ultimate solution. There seems to be a rush from family members, regardless of where they may be in the world, to the bedside before the patient dies. In other words, dying can offer a platform to make things better (say sorry, goodbye and share intimate details). However, this is not denying that the same platform can be used negatively by creating bitter arguments and disagreements. This seems more pronounced when there are money-related issues.

Some marriage ceremonies are brought forward in the face of death; this may arguably have a positive impact at different levels, physical, psychological, social and spiritual. Such marriages can take place at the bedside, which in essence involves the organisational system within health care to revolve around the dying patient. The catalyst for this may be the sudden realisation that time is short and everything has to be hurried and brought forward.

The knowledge that someone is dying tends to carry with it the attitude that they deserve the best of everything. For example, governments and charities dedicate their time and money to providing the best possible care for the dying (the latter relying on the generosity of the donations received to support their respective organisational vision). A diagnosis of cancer often carries an internal driver and emotive connotations for lay carers and the general public. This explains the underlying philanthropic approach in most western societies.

Palliative-care provision has been transformed by the introduction of the World Health Organisation's (WHO) principles that guide standards worldwide. The expectation from these principles is that care is standardised to provide high-quality service for dying patients and their families. Admittedly, the professionals tend to determine the minimum standards, which may, in reality, be alien to some patients. The quality of the food, care, treatment and surroundings is often high in specialist palliative-care settings in comparison to other establishments.

Those patients who have been lonely may find themselves surrounded by healthcare professionals attending to their needs and wishes, and giving them special attention and respect. For example, care can be provided in their own home free of charge in the UK with extra support during the night. Therefore, one could argue that the process of dying may provide opportunities and possibilities that would have not been feasible beforehand.

If the assertions above are acceptable, patients with cancer as a diagnosis could be perceived as the 'advantaged dying' (see *Chapter 2*). Therefore, it could be argued that those patients dying from a non-cancer disease become the 'disadvantaged dying'. Such a discrepancy cannot be acceptable when the outcome (death) is the same, and may have a bearing on the bereavement process of relatives.

Death and the role of funeral directors

Following death, one wonders what influences the funeral director's choice of car to transport the dead body to the funeral service. More often than not, this is a hearse, a type of luxurious limousine, the likes of which some of the deceased might never have ridden in before. In comparison to health care, this would not equate to individualised care and therefore questions the thinking behind this practice. Interestingly, this historical tradition remains important despite changing attitudes and practices with the introduction, for example, of 'green' funerals and woodland burials (www.uk-funerals.co.uk/green-funerals.html).

It is true that relatives may not have a choice outside what is being offered by the funeral director. Nyatanga (2001) has argued that because of the apparent death-denial attitude in our society, not many people will go 'window shopping' for their coffin or funeral transportation. In most cases, these arrangements are left to the relatives after the patient has died. It is often difficult to disentangle practical arrangements and emotional distress, and they may be persuaded to buy funeral packages without scrutiny, choice or cost implication.

The power of death

It seems that some deaths give authorities such as governments the impetus, rationale and justification to introduce new and stringent laws. For example, the deaths as a result of the September 11th terrorist attacks in the USA in 2001 seem to have changed the way the USA relates to the rest of the world. War, executions, assassinations and bombings such as those in Bali in 2003 and Madrid in 2004 left great carnage and devastation. The impact of these atrocities has been multi-faceted, including suffering, depleted relationships, retaliation and the tightening of policies with regard to broadcasting, media reporting and security. Simply, people's lives have been changed by such events.

The deaths described above are slightly different in context from those encountered in palliative care, but perhaps remind us of the impact that death can have, not only on those left behind but also on society at large. The advent of accessible images of death such as beheadings, shootings and explosions as they occur, via television and the internet, may have lessened the impression that death is a natural process, so it is imperative that palliative-care providers strive to ensure that the final image of death is one that may ease the process of grief for the bereaved.

The irony of death-denial

There is an apparent dichotomy between the conscious and subconscious mind with regard to death. Whilst on a subconscious level, people continue to deny their inevitable demise, they are, however, consciously aware of the need to plan for or organise their post-death provision. For example, purchasing life assurance and funeral policies will help pay for their funeral service. In addition, writing and re-writing wills and the creation of 'memory boxes' may help perpetuate their memory. However, such overt preparations suggest that people may be aware that they will die one day, but may not always be willing to discuss this openly with loved ones (Glaser and Strauss, 1965).

Conscious thoughts sustain the knowledge that death is a certainty and are therefore 'pushed' to the subconscious until the person is faced with a life-limiting illness, when such thoughts may be drawn to the fore. But, for some, this is a struggle and they may prefer not to acknowledge that they are dying.

There is an irony here, as these two thought-processes compete throughout an individual's lifetime. This may create tension between the reality of the situation (impending death) and the power of the subconscious (death-denial). It is here that health professionals can play a crucial part in helping the patient reconcile the two. However, should the professional carer have a similar dichotomy, it may perpetuate the patient's death-denial tendency. Similarly, relatives may experience individual or parallel avoidance of reality, so in specialist palliative care it is the quality of the death that influences the way relatives negotiate their grief.

References

George R, Sykes A (1997) Beyond cancer? In: Clarke D (ed) *New Themes in Palliative Care*. Buckingham: Open University Press

Glaser BG, Strauss AL (1965) *Awareness of Dying*. Chicago: Aldine

Nyatanga B (2001) *Why is it so Difficult to Die?* London: Quay Books

Street A (1995) *Nursing Replay*. Edinburgh: Churchill Livingstone

Van Gennep A (1961) *The Rites of Passage*. Chicago: University of Chicago Press

www.uk-funerals.co.uk/green-funerals.html (accessed 1/10/04)

Index